This book is do [donated to]
Morrill Memorial Library
by the author upon a
request by a patron of the
library. June 12, 2007

A Long Goodbye
and Beyond

Coping with Alzheimer's

D0890624

Linda M. Combs

BookPartners
Wilsonville, Oregon

Cover design by Richard Ferguson
Text design by Sheryl Mehary

BookPartners, Inc.
P.O. Box 922
Wilsonville, Oregon 97070

To Mama, Daddy, and David
for their love and support

Contents

Acknowledgments

Thanks to my publisher, BookPartners, for their faith in this project.

Thanks to my editors, Thorn and Ursula Bacon, for helping to bring order, clarity, and focus to my manuscript.

Thanks to Sheryl Mehary for organizing and designing the text.

Thanks to Tom Novak for the illustrations.

Thanks to Jini Guti for marketing the book.

Thanks to Van Speros for administration.

Thanks to Betsy DeGraff for her administrative assistance.

Thanks to Jeanette McHone for originally suggesting that I put these experiences and frustrations on paper—and assuring me that my experiences would help others.

Thanks to Garlene Grogan for her special assistance.

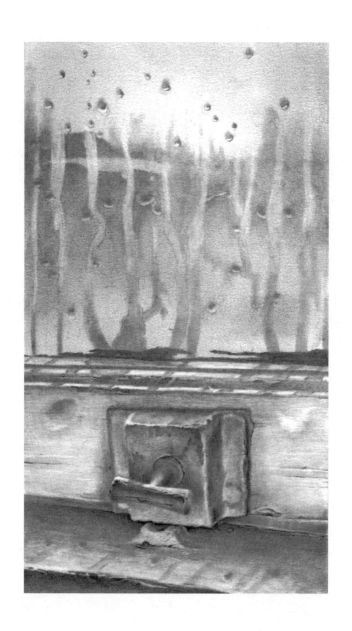

Introduction

As I look out the window each morning and see the sun glittering on the window pane or rain pattering on the glass, I realize once again how fortunate I am to be able to enjoy the moment—appreciate a sunrise, go for a walk, or enjoy a tasty breakfast. Every moment is precious, and I trust that the moments we spend together here in this book will be positive ones for you as well.

From time to time we all find ourselves trying to work through difficult and complex challenges in our lives. That's what this book is all about. I hope you will learn from and benefit by the experiences I reveal here, for you probably wouldn't be reading my words unless you or someone you know is affected by Alzheimer's disease. Thousands of families are involved with the "Curse of Forgetfulness"...the designation I have given to the malady that has struck the women and men in my family. And I...inheritor of the ancestral genes for intelligence, straight limbs and proud mind from my grandmother and mother...What of me? Will I, too, become a victim? There lies the question that haunts me, as I lie in my early morning bed, my husband gently asleep beside me. With my eyes closed, I listen to the morning sounds, identifying the birds by their cheerful wake-up calls, and hear the drowsy voice of the neighborhood traffic...and I wonder.

Chapter One

A Disease with a Past

~ ~

Alzheimer's—a terrifying, emotionally devastating word. When I used to hear it said, my palms instantly started to sweat, my breathing grew rapid, and a heaviness settled in the bottom of my stomach—almost as if I were going to erupt, or explode. I've never gotten used to the word because it has deep, unhappy meaning for me—awful meaning.

Alzheimer's is a most misunderstood disease.

A little learning is a dang'rous thing...
Alexander Pope
1688–1744

More and more people are beginning to grasp the terrible meaning associated with the word Alzheimer's. Four million people in the United States are now stricken with the disease. By the turn of the century five million people will be stricken, and within the next twenty years twelve million Americans are expected to lose their minds to this scourge. This year alone one hundred thousand people will die from the disease that is the fourth leading cause of death in the United States.

Why should I be so fearful and resentful of this disease? It stole my mother.

Ah, if you only knew the peace there is in an accepted sorrow.
                                        Jeanne de la Motte-Guyton
                                                    1648–1717

In my family, the disease has a history of claiming one relative after another for more than fifty years. Yes, I am a veteran of struggle with Alzheimer's. I know what it feels like to witness the deterioration of mind and body. I know how loving family members desperately try to help the victim in their custody, but what is there to do?

My strategy, defense, and attack is to direct my outrage into learning more about the disease and promising treatments.

Reading maketh a full man.

Francis Bacon
1561–1626

Even before an official diagnosis, fear and anxiety run rampant. The question arises, am I overreacting to what I see in this family member? Am I trying very hard to see things as normal when they are not normal? What is normal anyway? Still, the questions keep coming: Do all other families live like this? Has the afflicted person always behaved idiosyncratically and am I just now noticing what appears to be strange in her? Am I acting like she is myself? Would anyone tell me if I were? I hope that I will never have this disease, but I fear for myself and my family that the disease is lurking in my bloodstream waiting for the proper moment, when I have let my guard down, to spring.

We speak of hope; but is not hope only a more gentle name for fear?

Letitia E. Landon
1802–1838

Then, finally tests rule out other possible causes—and here come the fearful words—Alzheimer's disease—or probable Alzheimer's disease. What kind of terrible genes are we carrying to cause this attack? Is our family being punished? What are we supposed to learn from all of this pain? Are we too dense to "get it the first time"? Wouldn't one family victim be enough? How many more will there be? Is there something contagious in our environment—where we grew up—where my family lived? Frustrated, haunted by an enemy I cannot see, I embark on an investigation of the scourge. I am bold, angry, yet fearful, that my quest for knowledge and understanding of the reasons for the pain that has been visited on my family might awaken a more virulent strain of the disease, if there is such a thing. Don't forget, I tell myself, overcoming superstition is part of your search. In the years of the Black Plague in Europe, that disease was blamed on everything from witches to the evil eye of the moon in its first phase.

There is no cure for Alzheimer's disease. Will there ever be?

Nothing is so dear and precious as time.
Frances Rabelais
1494–1553

The causes of Alzheimer's disease are not known.

God is our refuge and strength, a very present help in trouble.
Psalms 46:1

Looking back, there were a number of early signs that indicated that Mother had Alzheimer's. Personality changes brought on sudden feelings of unexplainable unhappiness. Frequent crying was one of the ways in which her behavior changed. Her mood could change very rapidly from happy to sad, or sad to happy. She lost interest in sewing, something she had previously enjoyed a great deal. She had difficulty doing routine familiar tasks, such as setting the table for a meal. She sometimes became concerned about where she was and what time it was. She usually wanted to stay home, or go back home. She showed decreased judgment and diminished thinking skills when unfamiliar situations arose and decisions needed to be made. She was unable to "reason things out" as she had once been able to do so well. While she did not often actually lose things, she spent a great deal of time wondering where things were and working feverishly to locate them.

There is absolutely no cure or procedure to prevent the disease.

Seek the Lord and his strength: seek his face evermore.
Psalms 105:4

Senility, dementia, Alzheimer's: how are these conditions different?

Alzheimer's disease is the most common form of dementia in the United States. Dementia is often used to describe the loss of ability to reason, think, or remember.

Senility generally refers to mental weakness usually associated with old age—and it is often used interchangeably with "dementia." Alzheimer's is a progressive disease and its symptoms grow worse as time passes, and become more severe and more frequent.

The prognosis for development of Alzheimer's disease can be anything from two to more than twenty years. Many people believe that two to eight years after medical diagnosis is the span of time an afflicted person may be expected to live. However, this prediction must be modified by how quickly or how slowly the disease advances and how severe it is at the time of diagnosis.

Dwelling on how long this long goodbye will last is not useful. What is useful is a strong determination to make the best of whatever time is left.

I will say of the Lord, he is my refuge and my fortress: my God; in him will I trust.
Psalms 91:2

Each year we learn more and more about Alzheimer's. There are many dedicated scientists who are committed to learning about the progression of this disease. As they study possible ways to intervene or eventually prevent this disease, breakthroughs will be made. We need to know more about when the disease begins. Does it start up in the brain, for example, many years before it actually becomes evident through personality and behavioral changes? More research is currently being conducted to determine the answer to this question. Research findings may eventually lead to new and early-in-life diagnosis for Alzheimer's disease. If this happens, it might be possible to find ways to prevent or delay the ruinous development of the disease—and to do so before brain cells actually begin to die.

Other research focuses on ways to prevent the actual onset of the disease. This could be done if ways are found to protect the brain cells from being attacked by the scourge.

With my mother, disease has already been evident for more than twenty-three years. So, we wonder how long it will last.

My days are like a shadow that declineth; and I am withered like grass. But thou, O Lord, shalt endure for ever...

Psalms 102:11–12

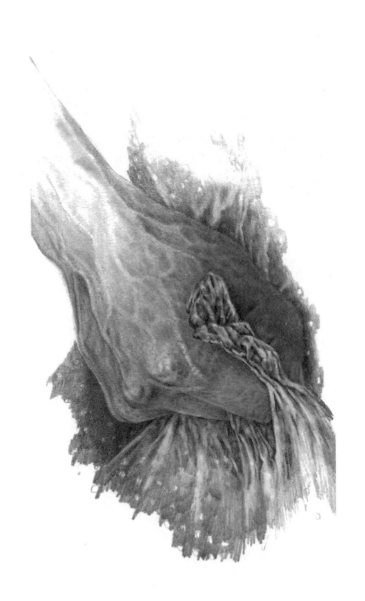

Chapter Two

My Personal Odyssey

~ ~

1950–1956

My personal odyssey with Alzheimer's began in about 1950. I remember when I was four years old, my maternal grandmother began doing strange things. She mumbled and babbled, became incontinent, burned her handmade pillowcases in the fireplace, and constantly twisted the skirt of her dress. All of these characteristics I recognize now as most likely symptoms of Alzheimer's. What I noticed as a child was that my mother brought more and more of the food for the traditional Sunday meal at my grandmother's, as Grandma prepared fewer and fewer of the wonderful dishes for which she was known. When Grandma let her, Mama spent most of Sunday afternoon combing the knots out of Grandma's hair, or cutting them free. Grandma never combed her hair between our visits.

By the time I was ten, Grandma was dead. During the six years before she died, my mother, some of Mama's sisters, and Grandpa had to care for Grandma. Almost every week on the way home from Grandma's, Mama would look at me and say, "Now, Linda, if something like this ever happens to me, please 'put me away' in an insane asylum. I do not want you to go through what I'm going through with my mama."

Mama didn't have a name for the illness Grandma had, but we all knew it was a horrible, powerful, and emotionally wounding disease, and that it affected our entire family—not just Grandma. Alzheimer's disease caused a condition of deteriorated mentality that eventually led to death.

> *Thou know'st 'tis common;*
> *all that live must die*
> *Passing through nature to eternity.*
>
> Shakespeare
> 1564–1616

1956–1974

Following Grandma's death, Grandpa and Mama would sometimes discuss some of the fond memories they had of Grandma. Grandpa usually concluded his part of the discussion with a puzzled look and said, "I don't know what happened to her, but for several years before she left this earth, she was 'crazier than a June bug.'" Mama seldom talked to me about

Grandma's final years, but chose instead to talk about the good times in our own family life. At this point she really seemed to make an even more determined effort to focus on our immediate family. Mama really knew how to make every day special—and how to make me feel special every minute we were together. In fact, she did this for everyone. When she walked into a room, suddenly everyone felt better just because she was there. This was a wonderful gift she had, and a part of her legacy I shall always cherish.

When better cherries are not to be had,
We needs must take the seeming best of bad.
Samuel Daniel
1562–1619

1975–1979

When Mama was fifty-one years old she began to exhibit some very vague signs of personality changes—feelings easily hurt, withdrawal from some social settings, and forgetting names of some acquaintances. These were all so vague, I chose to ignore them. At least, on most occasions I chose to ignore the changes. But after spending Thanksgiving with Mother and Daddy in 1975, I was brought to tears on the way home as I found the courage to discuss some of Mama's lapses with my husband, David. What was wrong with Mama? I couldn't pinpoint it.

To be conscious that you are ignorant is a great step to knowledge.
Benjamin Disraeli
1804–1881

We both were convinced that what we were observing was related to physical and emotional changes going on in her life at the time. Mama gradually lost her mind. I often chose to ignore her lapses because I didn't want to believe anything was wrong.

Hope springs eternal in the human breast.
Alexander Pope
1688–1744

I sometimes allowed myself to think back about Grandma during these times of reflection and wondered about what was wrong. I loved Mama so much that I didn't dare draw a parallel between her symptoms and what Grandma went through.

When my deep feeling of love for Mama did not appear to be strong enough to sustain me through the difficult times, I reminded myself of the strength and optimism she expressed during her own mother's illness.

Out of the lowest depths there is a path to the loftiest heights.
Thomas Carlyle
1795–1881

Where did all this strength and optimism come from? Mother was a very committed Christian. She accepted things for the way they were, while at the same time doing all that she could to make them better. Mama's attitude was courageous, proving her inner strengths, which resisted the disease as long as possible.

The Lord is my light and my salvation; whom shall I fear? The Lord is the strength of my life; of whom shall I be afraid?

Psalm of David 27:1

Mama knew that her strength came from the Lord, and that by relying on the fountainhead of her strength, she could change the way she felt about much that was going on in her life and around her. As a child, I observed her strength and commitment. Even then I realized that I could also change the way I felt about my circumstances in life. She left me this legacy and it gives me inspiration even today.

It seems to me we can never give up longing and wishing while we are thoroughly alive. There are certain things we feel to be beautiful and good, and we must hunger after them.

George Eliot
1819–1880

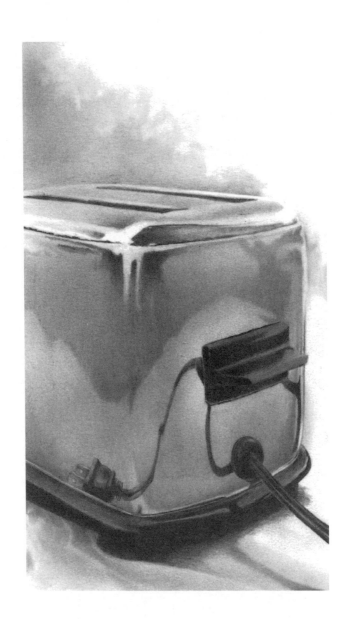

1980–1982

I noticed additional changes in Mama. When preparing to leave the house, she would check the stove many times to be sure all the burners were off. She always made sure her keys were in a special place each time in her purse, checking for them over and over again. She began to unplug every appliance in the house prior to leaving—TV, lamps, washing machine— everything. She stopped following recipes, saying that she just wanted to change some ingredients and do them her way. She made a lot of errors in her checkbook. She made a lot of corrections when she addressed envelopes, and the normal weekly letters she wrote to me when I was away became less and less frequent. During visits, her hugs and kisses were given infrequently. Mama wasn't responding as warmly and confidently to hugs and kisses as she traditionally had, but I never doubted that her love for me was still there.

Holy as heaven a mother's tender love, the love of many prayers and many tears which changes not with dim declining years.

Caroline Norton
1808–1877

Mama's illness drastically changed her life, thus causing her to bear a tremendous burden, but her courageous attitude was an inspiration to all of our family

The spirit of a man will sustain his infirmity; but a wounded spirit who can bear?

Proverbs 18:14

Mama loved creating beautiful things—delicate embroidery on pillowcases, original-design crochet ornaments, and handmade dresses. In 1982, Mama lovingly crocheted twenty afghans of various colors and presented them as gifts to me, my husband, and to other relatives. As mother was creating these lovely gifts, Alzheimer's disease was creating a painful process, a slow death, a very long funeral.

Talk happiness. The world is sad enough without your woe. No path is wholly rough. Look for the places that are smooth and clear, and speak of them to rest the weary ear of earth, so hurt by one continuous strain of mortal discontent and grief and pain.

Ella Wheeler Wilcox
1855–1919

1983–1985

The doctor ordered a battery of tests, but the tests showed nothing abnormal. Mama was not Mama anymore. She was not the mother I once knew. I loved her still.

Love is the life of the soul. It is the harmony of the Universe.
William Ellery Channing
1780–1842

Mama complained of feeling "crawly" things in her hair and asked me to look at her scalp and see if I could find anything wrong. What I saw was her beautiful hair. What she thought she felt was something else. Even today I love the memory I have of Mama. I love her for who she was. I'm unhappy for the person she has become. I've continued to love Mama and the person she has become. But, so often, I still ask myself, "Mama where are you?"

'Tis the mind that makes the body rich.
Shakespeare
1564–1616

Mama was known to her neighbors, friends, and relatives for her baking—home baked pies, cakes, and breads. She always enjoyed cooking and eating, but during this time she eliminated more and more foods from her table for one reason or another.

> *Not in the clamor of the crowded street*
> *Not in the shouts and plaudits of the throng,*
> *But in ourselves are triumph and defeat.*
>   Henry Wadsworth Longfellow
>   1807–1882

Cherry Blossom Festival
Washington, D.C., 1983

Mama was withdrawn and detached. Our lifetime of being a family unit—Mama, Daddy, Linda, and my husband, David— was coming to an end because Mama was leaving us; a little more of herself was disappearing each day. How can I explain the horror I felt? Think of a beautiful sculpture which gradually erodes before your eyes.

> *With all my will, but much against my heart, we two*
> *now part.*
>   Coventry Patmore
>   1823–1896

In 1984, when my swearing-in ceremony as Deputy Under Secretary for Management, United States Department of Education was held at the Department of Education in

Washington, D.C., Mama and Daddy came to be with me on that special day. My husband, David, and friends and relatives from North Carolina were there for the event, and Washington friends as well. Mother's social graces were still intact, and she enjoyed all of the events surrounding these occasions—except eating. She found almost nothing she could eat. According to her, her family doctor had informed her almost every food was not good for her for one reason or another. Her diet consisted of potatoes, vanilla ice cream, pound cake, and bread—all white foods—no color—no variety. I was sorry this was happening, and I thought it strange, but again, I found it easy to ignore. So, we had a wonderful time enjoying all the sights of Washington together.

> *It is the mind that maketh good or ill,*
> *That maketh wretch or happy, rich or poor.*
>   Edmund Spenser
>   1552–1599

I noticed when the 1985 Christmas Day photos were developed, Mama was not smiling in any of them. This was one of the times I felt helpless and heartbroken that I couldn't make Mama herself again. I wanted Mama to be able once again to celebrate birthdays with us, enjoy a family Thanksgiving dinner the way we used to, sing a hymn in church, or play "pull the string" with my cat. Mama was somewhat like a lovely vase with cracks in the surface that deepened every day. At some point, I knew the cracks would open wide and she would fall apart.

*If I can stop one heart from breaking, I shall not live
in vain.*

Emily Dickinson
1830–1886

1986

One day in June, Mama and I went shopping. We went to
a new shopping center where she had never been before. When
we arrived, she looked around and remarked, "It sure has been
a long time since I've been here." I gently reminded her that
this was a new place, that she and I had never visited. She made
the same comment five or six times during the course of our
three-hour excursion.

I knew something was wrong with Mama but continued to
hope there wasn't. She could not remember what had happened
to her just ten minutes ago.

*However deceitful hope may be, yet she carries us
on pleasantly to the end of life.*

La Rochefoucauld
1613–1680

On that same day she bought me a birthday present, which
I tried on in the store. She paid for it, had it wrapped, gave it to
me, and asked me to open it at a time nearer to my birthday. On

the way home she asked me at least eight times, "Now, did I get you anything for your birthday?"..."Now, did I get you anything for your birthday?"...That's when I knew something was very wrong. Mama did too. Quite often she would say, "I sure hope I'm not getting like my mama." I hoped that too. Mama was conducting herself the way Alzheimer's disease compelled her to, not the way she chose to conduct herself.

> *Confusion now hath made his masterpiece.*
>   Shakespeare
>   1564–1616

On one occasion I said to her, "Well, Mama, do you really think you are getting like Grandma?" She didn't answer. I'll never know whether she had reached the point where she could not follow a conversation to its logical conclusion, or whether it was just too painful for her to discuss. Her self-confidence was shattered. Her trust and belief in herself were gone.

> *Soon there will be nothing left with which to compare myself.*
>   Lady Ise
>   875–938

The battery of tests that had been done on Mama three years previously suddenly had more meaning. They had shown nothing, yet the evidence of her deterioration was right here before my eyes. Alzheimer's could not be positively confirmed, but other diseases were now ruled out and the clinical diagnosis was "probable Alzheimer's." Changes in her brain caused changes in her disposition.

To something new, to something strange.
Henry Wadsworth Longfellow
1807–1882

Mama always had wonderful taste in clothing. She sewed for herself and for me, and fashioned many handmade garments that fit perfectly. In these garments, all the seams were finished, buttonholes were bound, and hem tape was meticulously applied. When she shopped for ready-made clothing, she looked for clothing with these same refinements. Beginning about 1985 she purchased clothing for herself that did not fit properly and was of sub-standard fabrication, improperly sewn.

At other times Mama did familiar things and appeared to be the same person, but she wasn't.

Familiar acts are beautiful through love.
Shelley
1792–1822

Sometimes all I could think about was how much I wanted Mama to be Mama again—if only for a brief moment.

The sweet expression of that face,
Forever changing, yet the same.

Samuel Rogers
1763-1855

When was the last time you really had an uninterrupted two-hour interval to think about your own life—appreciate the life around you—accept yourself and your circumstances for what they are—and reach for more and more strength? I did when I drove from my home to my parents' home. Mama occupied my thoughts most of the time. I prayed for strength and patience.

Let prayer be the key of the morning and the bolt of
the evening.

Matthew Henry
1662–1714

This two-hour introspection and conversation with myself went on several times a month for years and years. Sometimes there would be something funny to chuckle about—other times the sadness would be overwhelming. I'd often have thoughts of happy times with Mama. I'd treasure and admire those thoughts and then put them away for a while. Those were some special memories, and they'd make me feel contented.

Life consists of what a man is thinking of all day.
Ralph Waldo Emerson
1803–1882

But with each one of these trips I was more sure that we were truly dealing with our own long goodbye.... It was so sad to see Mama deteriorate and to endure the disappearance of our home life and family activities. I often reminded myself of how fortunate I was to have a caring husband. He endured my sadness with me.

Neither the sun or death can be looked at steadily.
La Rochefoucauld
1613–1680

1988

Mama looked at the newspaper for an hour, but she couldn't discuss anything she read. She couldn't put a meal together so that it would all get on the table at the same time. She had very little power to bring order to her life. Her entire life was disordered.

Order is the sanity of the mind, the health of the body, the peace of the city, the security of the state. As the beams to a house, as the bones to the microcosm of man, so is order to all things.
Robert Southey
1774–1843

She was confused about the month, day, and year. She was unable to give directions to her home where she and Daddy had lived for over forty years. She could not name roads, streets, or the town where I lived. Even though she wanted to, she could not do better. Sometimes she cried because her capacities were more and more diminished.

I wept for memory.
Christina G. Rosetti
1830–1894

She was not able to reason things out. She had difficulty understanding what she was reading. She could not sit down and talk pleasantly and leisurely as she once had done.

What's more miserable than discontent?
Shakespeare
1564–1616

Her days of organized housework, gardening, and other pleasurable activities were disorganized. Much of what she thought she was doing did not get done at all.

Mama frenetically paced around the house and was unable to sit still. It must have broken Mama's heart to realize that the life she loved was disappearing around her. She had so looked forward to unstructured time for her creative projects such as her handwork, cooking, and gardening. Her world had revolved around love of home and family.

We will never have a better home,
if my opinion stands,
Until we commence a-keepin' house,
in the house not made with hands.

Will Carleton
1845–1912

She could not name the job I had or talk about what I did. She had difficulty engaging in conversation. She could talk only about the things she could do herself, such as a detailed description of how to crochet or how to bake a cake.

Mama was agitated and restless. She could not sit down at the table long enough to eat a meal without getting up several times.

I am condemned to a feverish unrest.
Marceline Desbordes-Valmore
1786–1859

She told the same stories over and over again, always about something that happened long ago, but never about anything that happened yesterday or today. Mama's retreat to her new world took place one tiny step at a time, day after day.

My heart is heavy at the remembrance of all the
miles that lie between us; and I can scarcely believe that
you are so distant from me. We are parted; and every

parting is a form of death, and every reunion is a type of heaven.

Johathan Edwards
1703–1758

She would often reflect on achievements in her professional life in the insurance business, or moral dilemmas that she had experienced relative to working versus staying at home. She would talk about how difficult it was to do both and to feel that she was successful at both. I was always glad to hear her talk about those things and to hear her rationale and her philosophy. I have since hoped that she realized how valuable these discussions were to me. Mama slipped away—one teardrop after another.

Gather ye rosebuds while ye may,
Old time is still a-flying;
And that same flower that blooms today,
Tomorrow will be dying.

Herrick
1591–1674

Dialogue was more and more difficult for her, so her solution to that dilemma was to do a monologue. Then she came to rely on my Dad more and more to complete the monologue, and she would say, "Oh, Robert, tell them about..." This he would dutifully do. But the stories she asked him to complete became fewer and fewer, shorter and shorter. Once sensible and serene, she was now confused and agitated.

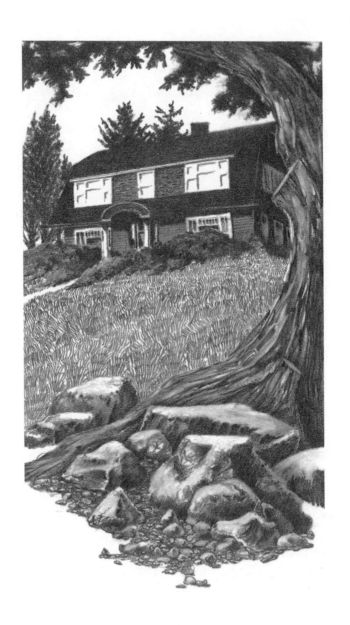

*A contented mind is the greatest blessing a man can
enjoy in this world.*

Joseph Addison
1672–1719

More than ever, Mama cooked, baked, and prepared less
and less food. Her daily diet continued to be quite unusual:
oatmeal, potatoes, and pound cake. Daddy was preparing most
of the meals at this point. However, he never told me this until
much later. When we went home to North Carolina to visit,
there would be those wonderful chocolate and coconut cakes,
pound cakes, chocolate pies—just like Mama always used to
make prior to our arrival. Later I learned that Daddy was the
one who oversaw the preparation—measuring all the ingredients himself, but letting Mama do what she could to put them
together. What a devoted, loving husband he was, to help Mama
continue to preserve her dignity and purpose for as long as she
could. But eventually, as her logical thinking process continued
to deteriorate, attempting to reason with her did not work.

*...(the) truth is my poor mind is so weak that I
never dare trust my own judgment in anything. What I
think one hour in a fit of low spirits makes me unthink
the next.*

Mary Anne Lamb
1764–1847

Mama wandered all through the house and was never still. She asked the same monotonous questions over and over again. She repeated the same household chores. She was preoccupied with keeping things clean and in place. One spot of water on the cabinet was wiped up with a paper towel immediately. A single glass in the sink had to be washed. She did laundry each day. She folded facial tissues and hoarded them in drawers for safe-keeping. She reorganized her drawers over and over again, neatly folding her gowns, underclothes, and pantyhose. Her actions were changeable and uncertain.

> *Life may change, but it may fly not;*
> *Hope may vanish, but can die not;*
> *Truth be veiled, but still it burneth;*
> *Love repulsed, but it returneth!*
>
> Shelley
> 1792–1822

Often when we went home for a visit with Mama and Daddy we dined out at a restaurant. This seemed to be less stressful for all of us. Mama would often spot someone in a restaurant and say, "I haven't seen her for a long time," and sometimes she'd go over and start talking with the woman or the couple. Often they would not have any idea who she was, but in Mama's small town people were usually quite considerate and helpful, so they would be pleasant. Mama did not always realize what she was doing.

There never was anybody like me!
For always when I wish to behave best,
something or other comes across me...
                                        Joanna Baillie
                                        1762–1851

Mama couldn't stand to see anything out of place, or left open—even a shirt collar. In fact, she saw an unbuttoned shirt collar as an invitation to button it up—on herself or on anyone else whose collar offended her. One particular evening, during dinner in a restaurant, she spotted an open shirt collar on a gentleman at the table next to us. Before we knew it, she was talking with the gentleman and her hands were headed straight for his shirt collar. This lack of social graces was so unlike her.

There are people whose characters cannot be judged from their behavior in society.
                                        Germaine de Stael
                                        1766–1817

While I was able to maneuver Mama back into her chair at our table and offered apologies to the gentleman, I began to feel that maybe eating out wasn't much less stressful than dining at home. Following this incident, I began to carry along little business-card-sized notes that I could easily slip to others. These note cards, written in my own handwriting, merely said, "My mother is a victim of Alzheimer's." I hoped this would

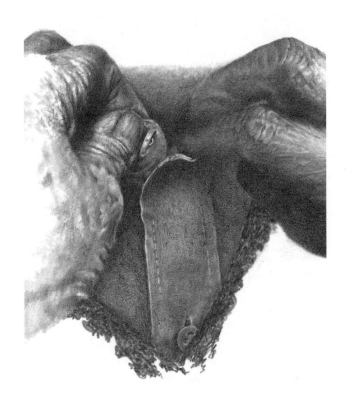

help me and others better understand that Alzheimer's is a sickness, not a shame.

> *The heart will break,*
> *yet brokenly live on.*

> Lord Byron
> 1788–1824

When others asked what was wrong with Mama, I answered by saying, "Mama is terminally ill. She has Alzheimer's disease." This helped me grasp the magnitude of her incurable illness.

> *All the best days of life slip away from us poor mortals and illness, dreary old age and pain sneak up, like mourners at the funeral of youth. Finally, with a fierce scowl, harsh death, who has come at last, snatches us away.*

> Virgil
> 70–19 B.C.

Back home, Mama followed Daddy around—from room to room in the house, into the garden, everywhere. She was always right beside him, especially when he was on the phone. So, there was virtually no opportunity for him to talk openly and freely to me about some of the difficult times he was having with Mama. Daddy was her only security in an increasingly confusing world. Mama's words and actions were dictated by her unsound mind. Her usual loving attitude was displayed less and less frequently.

> *I am not of revengeful temper, but have a childlike mind.*
>
> Sappho
> 610–635 BC

Mama stopped taking her medicine because she could not remember if she had already swallowed it. Daddy had to take over the task of administering her pills. Once solid as a rock, Mama was now confused, volatile, and unsettled.

> *Between two worlds life hovers like a star,*
> *'Twixt night and morn, upon the horizon's verge.*
>
> Lord Byron
> 1788–1824

1989

Mama's memory loss became worse and worse. Her changes were more obvious; as she became more confused, she began to neglect her personal care. She hid things such as her pocketbook or her car keys in unusual places—like the refrigerator. She was very suspicious of others. She sometimes accused others of stealing her personal belongings.

My peace is gone. My heart is heavy.

Goethe
1749–1832

She began to shuffle her feet as she walked, much as I had seen and heard Grandma do many years earlier. She was often agitated, irritable, quarrelsome, and improperly dressed. She was not intentionally being defiant. She could not help it.

One kind word can warm three winters.

Japanese proverb

It was so unpleasant, so difficult to deal with Mama's actions. How could I get beyond this? Although I did not like some things Mama did, that did not change my love for her.

Love is all we have,
The only way,
That each can help the other.

Euripides
408 B.C.

I realized that if I were ever going to get beyond this, I really needed to find a way to cope—a way that worked for me, to get rid of all those useless feelings. Sometimes I felt displeasure, but it was much more useful to replace that feeling with more loving thoughts of Mama.

Hide in your heart a bitter thought
Still it has power to blight
Think love, although you speak it not,
It gives the world more light.

Ella Wheeler Wilcox
1855–1919

Why was I sometimes angry, and with whom? What was I supposed to learn from this? How could I work through this and get beyond all this anger? This disease taught me a lot about self-discipline and control. It taught me that it takes a lot of energy to be angry.

If anger is not restrained, it is frequently more hurtful to us than the injury that provokes it.

Seneca
4 B.C.–65 A.D.

Mama was eating less than ever, and her weight dropped thirty pounds. Once sweet and charming, Mama was robbed, by sickness, of her sophistication, grace, and charm.

But were it to my fancy given
To rate her charms, I'd call them heaven.

Charles Dibdin
1745–1814

In September of 1989 I had another swearing-in ceremony. This one was at the Department of the Treasury in Washington, D.C., where I had been appointed by the President of the United States and confirmed by the United States Senate to be the Assistant Secretary for Management at the Department of the Treasury. But for this event, my biggest booster and supporter would not be there.

Mama's illness changed her from

- self-sufficient to dependent
- artistic to unimaginative
- serene to agitated
- tranquil to frenetic
- cheerful to shattered
- confident to disoriented
- expressive to emotionally detached
- inquisitive and intelligent to confused
- motivated to preoccupied
- meticulous to careless
- optimistic to anxious
- perceptive to senile
- polished to inarticulate
- self-confident to insecure
- loving to hostile and suspicious

It is a rare and difficult attainment to grow old gracefully and happily.
                                        Lydia M. Child
                                        1802–1880

I would talk by phone to Mama and Daddy a couple of times a week. I would hear from Daddy that there were some nights Mama could not sleep. My research on Alzheimer's and what I observed later confirmed what Daddy had said. I found it typical that Mama would get up and wander into the kitchen, and attempt to prepare a meal, or move things around and hide them.

Mama's good-natured spirit often displayed itself as an abusive spirit.

I once knew a man out of courtesy help a lame dog over a stile, and he for requital, bit his fingers.
                                        William Chillingworth
                                        1602–1644

Unless one has lived with this disease day in and day out, it is difficult to imagine how much energy must be spent by the caregiver and how much creativity must be applied each and every moment of the day and night. There is little if any peace for the caregiver. Every moment of Daddy's life was spent concerned about Mama.

Sometimes Mama attempted to do things that were unsafe. We tried to create safety without causing conflict.

Blessed are the happiness makers; blessed are they that remove friction, that make the courses of life smooth and the converse of men gentle.
Henry Ward Beecher
1813–1887

Even though Daddy began to flip the circuit-breaker switch in the power box when he went to bed at night, so that the electric stove could not be turned on, there were other concerns when darkness fell. Sometimes, Mama would awaken and he had a hard time getting her back into bed. Often, he was not successful and the two of them were up for long hours.

I recall that on Christmas morning in 1989, although we were all together as we usually were, I felt such sadness. We were together, but we weren't all there.

To lose a friend is the greatest of all losses.
Syrus
45 B.C.

I despaired that Mama could not sit still long enough to talk pleasantly and in a leisurely way, as we once did. But there was a sense of warmth just being with her.

A true friend is the greatest of all blessings.
                                        La Rochefoucauld
                                        1613–1680

Such sorrow and loneliness...I didn't want Mama to be leaving me.... I knew she didn't want to be leaving me either — but she was. I felt abandoned, almost orphaned.

> *Alone, on a wide, wide sea,*
> *So lonely 'twas that God himself*
> *Scarce seemed there to be.*
>
>   Coleridge
>   1772–1834

Such isolation. Such uncomfortableness. I understood, but...I disliked being isolated from family and friends. Many people were uncomfortable being around Mama, so they didn't visit very often.

> *He who cannot forgive others breaks the bridge over*
> *which he must pass himself.*
>
>   George Herbert
>   1593–1633

Alzheimer's is a family disease — I mean it has an impact on every member of the family. Family members need support as well as the victim. Often they require more health resources and suffer from an increased number of illnesses themselves.

This is probably due to the stress and anxiety being experienced by them over the progressive loss they see advancing in their loved one. Also, family members fear that what they observe in their afflicted loved one may someday come to visit them. And while many families lose control of the family life, others are pulled together by this illness.

Each one of us has a choice of becoming better or bitter from dealing with this disease.

> *Let the words of my mouth and the meditation of my heart be acceptable in thy sight, O Lord, my strength, and my redeemer.*
>
> Psalms 19:4

There are a number of things I've learned from other families that have caused them to become better and not bitter as they deal with this long goodbye. Trying to pull a family together can sometimes be challenging, but if done in the right spirit, can often prove to be very rewarding. I found it difficult to talk about this disease at first, primarily because I didn't feel as though I had enough information. So, first of all, even before a medical diagnosis of Alzheimer's, or probable Alzheimer's, has been given, it would be a good idea to order some of the free information from the Alzheimer's Association. Then, following an official medical diagnosis, as the primary caregiver, a next step would be to invite family, dear friends, possibly close neighbors, and (if you feel it is appropriate) the Alzheimer's afflicted loved one to have a discussion session. Several families have told me that a discussion session is quite useful.

If many of the family members live out of town and cannot come to this initial discussion session, a conference telephone call is an alternative. It's best to tell everyone all together, but not imperative. Use your own good judgment about how to accomplish this.

Families who have done this say that the first thing to do is to tell everyone is about the medical diagnosis and explain what Alzheimer's actually is, using the free material from the Alzheimer's Association. Be candid about the fact that your Alzheimer's loved one will get worse, and give them one of the free brochures to take home with them. Explain what the physician has recommended and when the next medical appointment is to take place.

Explain some of the things the caregiver needs to do for the Alzheimer's loved one, and some of the things that will be needed in the future. Also make it clear that as the primary caregiver you will need help in determining just what is needed in this challenging situation. Everyone needs to be able to deal with this in the most positive way possible. In one way or another this disease will affect each family member and friend.

Families who have gone through this discussion session tell me that there is usually one member who speaks up to say that they can't help at all. Do not be alarmed by this statement. Instead, let the person know that while the disease has a deteriorating effect primarily on a specific member of the family, it also has an emotional effect on the entire family. Each family member or friend will not be comfortable doing the same things, but all can support one another in a positive way. The important point here is to keep alert to find the best ways to support each other.

If you are a family that prays together, a good conclusion to this session would be to read a comforting passage of scripture such as Psalm 23 and to close with a prayer.

The Lord is my shepherd; I shall not want.

He maketh me to line down in green pastures: he leadeth me beside the still waters.

He restoreth my soul: He leadeth me in the paths of righteousness for his name's sake.

Yea, though I walk through the valley of the shadow of death, I will fear no evil: for thou art with me; thy rod and thy staff they comfort me.

Thou preparest a table before me in the presence of mine enemies: thou anointest my head with oil; my cup runneth over.

Surely goodness and mercy shall follow me all the days of my life: and I will dwell in the house of the Lord for ever.

Psalm 23

After some time passes, caregivers have told me, it becomes obvious how family, friends, and neighbors are responding. So, having another discussion session in a few weeks or months is most appropriate. If things have not worked out as the caregiver had hoped, it's important to be honest about those concerns. Keep in mind that the ultimate goal of the caregiver is to establish the best quality of life possible for both the caregiver and the Alzheimer's loved one. This is most likely the goal of family and friends too, but sometimes they need some coaching in how to help. Families can be a real drain on the caregiver, or they can be a true source of support and help. Caregivers must learn to seek needed help and support from others—family, friends, and professionals.

> *Adversity is sometimes hard upon a man.*
> *But for one man who can stand prosperity, there are*
> *a hundred that will stand adversity.*
>
> Thomas Carlyle
> 1795–1881

As a caregiver, I have learned that I owe it to myself to take care of my own health and well-being. Periodically, I go through my own little checklist to see how I am doing. I ask myself if I am...

eating right,

getting enough rest,

finding time for prayer and study that give me needed strength,

having time with friends,
finding leisure time for things I enjoy,
feeling tension and pressure,
feeling a lot of conflict with my Alzheimer's loved one,
crying a lot,
permitting my own health or personal care to suffer,
feeling guilt and pain about this situation,
feeling inadequate to deal with this disease,
learning to find the blessings in my role as a caregiver,
worrying about financial burdens,
asking for help from family, friends, neighbors, or
    professionals,
attending a caregiver support group.

Answering these questions periodically helps me to keep a check on myself, and they make me more aware of the pressures and stresses I am feeling in my situation. I try to keep in mind that the health and care needs of Mama and Daddy, my current care receivers, will change. So, also, will the health and care needs of me as their caregiver change. My own physical and emotional well-being are very important.

But thou, Oh Lord, art a shield for me; my glory, and the lifter up of mine head.

Psalm 3:3

1990

Mama was not able to count money, dress herself, or perform other daily routine tasks without assistance from Daddy.

Adversity has the effect of eliciting talents, which in prosperous circumstances would have lain dormant.
                                        Horace
                                  65 B.C.–8 B.C.

As Daddy did more and more, Mama was able to do less and less. She drifted away.

A poor man served by thee, shall make thee rich
A sick man helped by thee, shall make thee strong
. Thou shalt be served thyself by every sense
Of service which thou renderest.
                          Elizabeth Barrett Browning
                                  1806–1861

Daddy said he prayed daily for God's will to be done with Mama, and he only asked one thing: that he be allowed to be well and strong enough to take care of Mama for as long as she needed him.

God give us grace
Each in his place
To bear his lot
And murmuring not,
Endure and wait and labor.

Martin Luther
1483–1546

I learned in phone conversations, and I could see when I came home for a visit, that this disease was continuing to further destroy the nature of Mother and Daddy's relationship—and of my relationship with this wonderful, talented woman. The disease was breaking up Mama and Daddy's home life. It was ruining all their plans for a full and complete retirement life. Mama and Daddy worked hard to build their life together and to have their special time together. Now all of that was evaporating.

Nothing that is can pause or stay;
The moon will wax, the moon will wane,
The mist and clouds will turn to rain
The rain to mist and cloud again,
Tomorrow be today.

Henry Wadsworth Longfellow
1807–1882

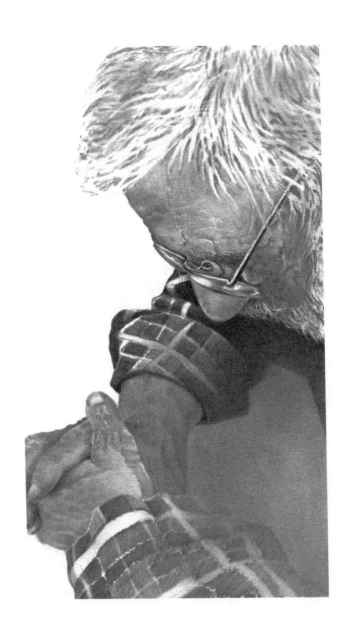

When I came home for visits, the difficulties with each and every situation during the day and night were just grueling. These times emphasized to me what my daddy was going through each and every moment of each and every day. Mama frequently tested my patience when she refused to do things I requested. One cold, wintry day when we were going out to eat, she refused to get into the car. She also refused to go back into the house.

It is the difficulties that show what men are.
Epictetus
50–120 A.D.

I could never predict what Mama was going to do. Sometimes she attempted to dress too warmly in summer and not warmly enough in winter.

I would not anticipate the relish of any happiness,
nor feel the weight of any misery,
before it actually arrives.
Joseph Addison
1672–1719

How shocked I always was when Mama came out with blatant refusals for the simplest of requests. Pleading, begging, and demanding did not work at all. In fact, it just made things worse.

And many a word at random spoken
May soothe, or wound, a heart that's broken
Sir Walter Scott
1771–1832

Sometimes asking pleasantly didn't work either. Sometimes it did.

Whatsoever ye would that men should do to you, do
ye even so to them.
Matthew 7:12

What worked one day didn't always work the next.

The sun shines after every storm;
there is a solution for every problem,
and the soul's highest duty is to be of good cheer.
Ralph Waldo Emerson
1803–1882

The chores associated with daily health habits were often such a source of frustration for me. Mama sometimes didn't brush her teeth and wouldn't let us help her brush them. This disappointed us, but we usually realized that it was more important to let her do things her way than to attempt to alter her life in ways that caused her discomfort or unhappiness.

Our actions, depending upon ourselves, may be controlled, while the powers of thinking, originating in higher causes, cannot always be moulded to our wishes.
George Washington
1732–1799

Mama did things that were so unlike her. As she lost some of her social graces, she did things I found distasteful, things that were shocking and revolting as she deteriorated slowly, inexorably, but I reminded myself the disease was dictating Mama's behavior, and it was up to me to show her my love despite her unlovable manners.

Act well at the moment, and you have performed a good action to all eternity.
Lavater
1741–1801

I constantly adjusted what I expected of Mama. I wished I had taken courses in drama and pantomime in college. "Showing her" instead of "telling her" was often most effective.

Our greatest glory is not in never failing but in rising every time we fall.
Oliver Goldsmith
1730–1774

My thoughts often revolved around what I could be doing. I often wondered if I could be doing more. We learned that just being with Mama seemed to make her the most comfortable.

It is the greatest of all mistakes to do nothing because you can only do a little. Do what you can.
Sydney Smith
1771–1845

Conversations during this time were often not conversations at all. Words or even sentences may have come forth from Mama, but she couldn't concentrate long enough to wait for a reply—or to understand one. I felt sad when Mama attempted to relate a past event, but could only remember a small portion of what she wanted to say. Sometimes she could concentrate long enough to be assisted with the story, but other times we were unable to help her.

The winds of sadness lay siege
To my forsaken mind, my wounded heart.
Kata Szidonia Petroczi
1662–1708

There were always tasks associated with daily living when Mama and I were together. I continued to be amazed that Daddy could actually go through these chores every day. Helping Mama bathe, supplying forgotten names, places, dates, days of the week, and answering the same questions over and over again became a natural, but very tiring routine.

> *Love me a little, love me long.*
> > Christopher Marlowe
> > 1564–1593

Mama presented a real challenge when her hair needed combing and shampooing, or when she needed a bath. She usually would not let anyone help her. Since she had no concept of time, she thought that she had just had a bath and shampooed her hair. In reality, several days may have passed between bathings.

> *An able man shows his spirit by gentle words and resolute actions; he is neither hot nor timid.*
> > Chesterfield
> > 1694–1773

I was sometimes needlessly exasperated trying to help Mama do things she didn't want to do.

> *It is by presence of mind in untried emergencies that the native mettle of a man is tested.*
> > James Russell Lowell
> > 1819–1891

Mama did not react reasonably. She was mentally unsound—not reasonable.

What can we reason, but from what we know?
Alexander Pope
1688–1744

Even though I was good, kind, and usually patient with Mama, I learned not to expect the same courtesies from her.

When you are good to others,
you are best to yourself.
Benjamin Franklin
1706–1790

It was always a creative challenge to find ways to keep Mama involved and useful. But Daddy and I became quite good at discovering small tasks around the house that she could do, especially the housework. Everything we attempted did not work out perfectly with Mama, but next time we just tried again, or tried a different way.

Last week I saw a man who had not made a mistake
in 4,000 years. He was a mummy in the British Museum.
H. L. Wayland
1796–1865

When I was with Mama, I learned to expect the unexpected.

What we anticipate seldom occurs; what we least expected generally happens.
                                        Benjamin Disraeli
                                        1804–1881

Visits to the doctor or dentist were challenging. Mama often refused to let us take her to the doctor or dentist. Many times we were powerless to help her.

Most powerful is he who has himself in his power.
                                        Seneca
                                        4 B.C.– 65 A.D.

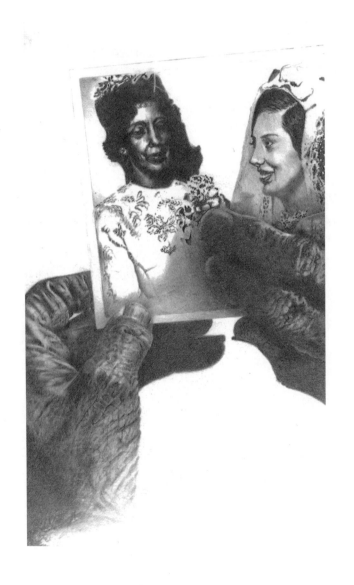

Chapter Three

Creating Advocates—Not Adversaries

~ ~

As we are going through the daily trials and tribulations of caregiving, we must continually find ways to create advocates or helpers—for our loved one as well as for ourselves. Often the family physician can be one of those sources.

During the long duration of Mother's illness, I have witnessed first-hand a number of physicians and how they deal with the patient, the caregiver, and other family members. A concerned, caring attitude demonstrates to the patient and family members that the physician will indeed be supportive. I look for signs or demonstrations of an attitude that seems to say, "We are in this together," or "I don't have all the answers, but we'll work through this together step by step."

Valuable is the physician who offers careful, systematic testing and a simple, direct explanation of the plan for diagnosis. It is helpful to know ahead of time that you, as the caregiver, will be asked to provide patient history, current patient information, drugs currently taken, diet, and special problems with the patient. When the physician discusses what will be done in terms of simple paper/pencil tests of cognitive ability, and explains even such things as simple reflex tests to the caregiver and the patient ahead of time, a tremendous weight of concern is lifted. If CAT, EEG, or other lab tests will be performed upon the initial visit, it is helpful to know that ahead of time as well. These discussions prior to beginning the initial diagnosis give a strong indication that the physician is a person who looks ahead and will inform patient and caregiver about procedures, because he or she knows it will be comforting.

Prior to the time of testing, the physician should prepare the caregiver and patient regarding the length of time the tests will take, how many office visits will be required, and over what period of time.

As caregiver, get an understanding ahead of time about how the "results session" will be conducted. Will it be conducted in person, with caregiver and patient, or will you get the results over the phone? If you as caregiver have a prefer-ence, you must express your desire.

The physician should be eager to share information about where the caregiver can go for additional help. At the least, toll-free numbers should be available for places where you can seek assistance after the condition is diagnosed. A physician who truly encourages caregivers and family members to seek emotional support from support groups, toll-free help lines, and internet sites is performing his or her duty at a very high service level. Physicians should not assume that they are responsible only for scientific diagnosis and treatment of the patient. They have a larger obligation—to act as a partner and advocate for the patient and the caregiver. One of the most positive things a physician can do to assist caregivers is to see the patient at the appointed time. This sounds so simple and unimportant unless you've ever been the victim of a long wait. A physician's waiting room can be a fearful place, especially for a demented patient. It can also be very trying to caregivers who must answer the patient's question every five minutes, "When are we going home?" or, "What am I doing here anyway?"

Upon seeing the patient and caregiver, the physician needs to talk about safety. Is it still permissible for the patient to drive? Are there safety hazards around the house such as rugs to trip over, appliances that can be left on and forgotten, or other hazards that could lead to a fall? The physician should make certain that the caregiver is aware that the safety of the patient is a priority.

There are other aspects of patient care for the physician to mention as well. Bringing to the attention of the caregiver the need to monitor such things as diet; rest; personal care; medication; changes in appetite and bladder and bowel functions; sitters and visiting nurses; meals on wheels; and other community services, is yet another display of support.

Physicians need to realize that the patient they see for twenty minutes may be "superficially normal" for that period of time. If memory problems are presented, the physician must listen carefully to see if the patient is evading direct questions, covering up, or letting the caregiver speak for the patient. If the physician would only multiply what he or she sees in that twenty minute office visit by seventy-two, a much greater appreciation would be guaranteed of what the caregiver is going through each day. (Seventy-two reflects the number of twenty-minute segments the caregiver is spending with the patient each and every day.)

A physician should talk about possibilities, probabilities, and certainties regarding the diagnosis. For example, some dementia is reversible and treatable. Some can be slowed or halted, but most cannot. This discussion begins a process that can help prepare the patient and the caregiver for such a diagnosis. It is always important to help family members and caregivers feel that they have acted in a responsible manner by seeking a complete diagnosis. The physician should be willing to make referrals if the family or patient wishes them, or if the physician feels it would assist in making a better diagnosis.

The physician should let the family, caregiver and patient know that one of the goals of the physician is to work with them through this situation. A family is truly blessed when the physician becomes a sensitive and caring member of the family support team. If the diagnosis is positive for Alzheimer's disease, supportive statements such as, "Unfortunately things will get worse, but we can work through this together," can really mean a lot to a family member, caregiver, and patient.

Wise is the physician who is able to look at the total patient, not just the charts. Does this patient live alone? Does the patient have family support close by, or is long-distance caregiving taking place?

A few times I've encountered physicians who do or say things that make caregivers and family members feel uncomfortable or dissatisfied. "Nothing can be done," is one such statement. Maybe nothing can be done to change the diagnosis or cure the disease, but there are lots of other things that can be done to help caregivers, family members, and patients cope with Alzheimer's and its symptoms.

Most likely part of the reason for seeing a physician and seeking a diagnosis is that the patient is experiencing memory loss. Telling caregivers or patients that progressive forgetting is part of "normal aging" is not comforting, and neither is it true.

Physicians should be sensitive to the feelings of the patient and the caregiver. Talking only to the caregiver or family member when the patient is also present is rude and insensitive.

Each family is different. They possess differing strengths and weaknesses. Some families are better equipped physically and emotionally to deal with Alzheimer's disease than others. Sensitive physicians recognize these differences and adjust the advice they give as needed.

The physician does not shoulder the entire burden. There are many things that the patient, family member, and caregiver must do to assist the physician. In preparation for a visit to the doctor, it is important to collect all of the patient's medications in a bag and carry them to the appointment. This includes prescription medications as well as over-the-counter medications.

Ahead of this initial visit, family members and caregivers (and the patient if he/she is still able) should talk about family medical history, especially diseases in the family, and things that have claimed the lives of other deceased family members. What was the cause of death of the patient's parents and grandparents? Compare and make notes about what is causing the patient to need medical attention at this time. Is it a sudden decline or a progressive decline, and in what ways? The person accompanying the patient to the doctor will then be better prepared to report these facts on medical forms or in conversation with the physician.

It's important to know the type of physician being consulted. Is this physician a specialist, a family doctor, or a primary care physician? If the patient is seeing a family doctor or a primary care physician, it's important to remember that they are generalists and are looking for many different things. If the patient is experiencing dementia, the caregiver should be prepared to ask for a referral to a neurologist or a psychiatrist. It's important to be open and forthright with the doctor and other health care professionals.

Caregivers must assume many roles. From time to time, spokesperson and interpreter between the patient and doctor is a necessary role, but only when the patient is incapable.

The reality of the diagnosis and the disease is sometimes a bitter pill to swallow, as is accepting the limitations of the Alzheimer's patient. As the disease progresses, sometimes family members ask and expect the physician to make some of the tough decisions that really must be made by the caregiver or family members on behalf of the patient. There may not be any simple solutions for some of these tough issues. So, as loved ones, we must not demand quick, easy answers from the physician.

It's imperative to recognize that the physician is a very busy person and to be respectful of his or her time. One of the best ways I know to use the physician's time wisely is to be prepared for the office visit. Go with a list of questions or concerns, and be attentive to the answers given.

I find it useful to keep in mind that as a caregiver and a loved one of an Alzheimer's patient, I am always trying to find an advocate, not an adversary. I need as many advocates as possible—for the patient, family members, and for me as a caregiver.

As caregivers we must always remember that we cannot possibly supply all the care that our loved one ultimately needs. We must continually seek help from volunteers, organizations, professionals, and family members. The individuals and organizations we select to be a part of our vital support team can help to make our caregiving adventures blessed and rewarding experiences.

I can't change Mama's illness. I can only give some comfort and lots of love to her.

When you have accomplished your daily task, go to sleep in peace; God is awake.
Victor Hugo
1802–1885

1990

Up and down, sit down, stand up, walk through the house, find a speck of fuzz on the carpet, pick it up, pick up a book, move it to another table—lots and lots of motion—all the time. During visits to Mama and Daddy's home, I became tired just watching all of Mama's restless motion. How long could Daddy continue as her constant companion and caregiver?

*The truly brave are soft of heart and eyes,
And feel for what their duty bids them do.*
Lord Byron
1788–1824

Mother had such a beautiful way of dressing. Her friends used to tell her that she should be a fashion model. She was so tall, graceful, and always so well-groomed. It broke my heart to see Mama dress with pants, long gown, blouse, and sweater, all at the same time.

> *And nature gave thee, open to distress,*
> *A heart to pity, and a hand to bless.*
>
> Charles Churchill
> 1731–1764

Sometimes I felt shame and embarrassment, but I reminded myself that I had no control over Mama's behavior.

> *A man is as miserable as he thinks he is.*
>
> Seneca
> 5–65 A.D.

When unusual or unpleasant things happened, I worked through them the best that I could.

> *I can not sweep the darkness out, but I can shine it out.*
>
> John Newton
> 1725–1807

1991

Daddy cared for Mama, loved her, and was her constant companion. One night she awoke startled, looked at him and said, "Who are you? What are you doing in my bed?" They had been married forty-six years and this statement broke his heart.

With each passing day, we saw Mama fading away—a step back in time—a step away from today.

> *To everything there is a season, and a time to every purpose under heaven.*
>
> Ecclesiastes 3:1

Mama usually would not accept help with dressing, bathing, or personal care. She was not communicative. She refused to eat. She lost control of her bladder and bowels and she was unstable on her feet. The disease that first destroyed Mama's mind continually destroyed her body also.

> *It's easy enough to be pleasant*
> *When life flows by like a song*
> *But the man worth while*
> *Is the one who can smile*
> *When everything goes dead wrong.*
> *For the test of the heart is trouble*
> *And it always comes with the years,*
> *And the smile that is worth*
> *The praise of earth*
> *Is the smile that shines through tears.*
>
> Ella Wheeler Wilcox
> 1855–1919

1991

One day I got a phone call I'll never forget. It was from my father saying he was just overwhelmed. It seemed that Mama had refused help from the visiting nurse and had become belligerent. When the nurse left, she said that she would not return. That left my father feeling totally isolated, helpless, and overwhelmed. I stood there with that phone in my hand, looking over at the White House from my office window at the Treasury building, and said, "Dear Lord, why are you giving me these great opportunities here, yet I'm so needed back home?" Mama's disease had changed my life in ways that I could not have imagined.

Would you fashion for yourself a seemly life?
Then do not fret over what is past and gone;
In spite of all you may have left behind
Live each day as if your life had just begun.
                                        Goethe
                                        1789–1832

So, a couple of months later I resigned my position as Assistant Secretary for Management at the United States Department of the Treasury in Washington, D.C., to move back to North Carolina and take a new position. This new position didn't require a resume. It didn't require an interview process. Unlike several of my other jobs, this one didn't require a Senate confirmation hearing. This position didn't have an organizational chart or even a functional job description. It really didn't even have a job title—but we've come to know it as Caregiver.

Mama's life had been drastically changed—so had the way of life of the entire family.

> *I am not now*
> *That which I have been.*
>
> Lord Byron
> 1788–1824

This new position took me from testifying in congressional hearings to interpreting hand motions that meant, "I'd like a sandwich, please." Sometimes Mama's actions were puzzling.

> *I have striven not to laugh at human actions, not to*
> *weep at them, nor to hate them, but to understand them.*
>
> Baruch Spinoza
> 1632–1677

I went from being the chief financial officer for an organization with a nine billion dollar budget to deciphering a checkbook and paying bills for my mother and dad. Mama was not Mama anymore. She was not the mother I once knew. Mama's sickness grew worse. I love her still.

Life is the flower of which love is the honey.

Victor Hugo
1802–1885

I went from managing personnel in a department that had 175,000 employees worldwide, to managing one mother in pure agony, suffering from Alzheimer's and vanishing right before my eyes. Outside she looked the same, but inside she was very different.

A mother is a mother still,
The holiest thing alive.

Coleridge
1772–1834

I went from coping with a calendar of meetings and appointments every fifteen minutes to coping with isolation, loneliness, and a profound sadness. There was an open wound down deep in my heart. It was a feeling of emptiness, but not a total void. A little bit of Mama remained, but most of her was gone.

Youth fades; love droops;
the leaves of friendship fall.
A mother's secret love outlives them all.

Oliver Wendell Holmes
1809–1844

I went from managing people who were working on issues affecting the lives of virtually every segment of the population of the United States to managing health care workers on round-the-clock shifts feeding, bathing, and diapering someone living in a world that we were not allowed to be a part of any more. I knew that Mama's future was most likely to be hopeless and painful.

Men must pursue things which are just in the present, and leave the future to the divine Provident.
                                        Francis Bacon
                                        1561–1626

I went from conferring with folks whom we often called upon to "have all the answers," to working with those who had, for the most part, no good answers. These were caring people who were doing their very best to give the finest care possible, but we were all just coping. We all grieved each day as we watched the spirit of Mama disappear, piece by piece. Mama where are you? Mama was gone. When did we say goodbye?

Who ran to help me when I fell
And would some pretty story tell,
or kiss the place and make it well?
My mother.

                                        Ann Taylor
                                        1782–1866

Those who loved Mama were her shadow, protecting and shielding her every moment, day and night.

The daisy, by the shadow that it casts,
Protects the ling'ring dewdrop from the sun.
                                        Wordsworth
                                        1770–1850

Mama's illness had a profound impact on Daddy. Through it all, he was good, loving, and kind to Mama.

Goodness is beauty in its best estate.
                                        Marlowe
                                        1564–1593

Near Father's Day, 1991

Daddy and I left Mama at home with a sitter to take a ride in the country. He showed me the two cemetery plots he had bought for them. He was preparing for the final goodbye.

Golden lads and girls all must like chimney sweepers, come to dust.
                                        Shakespeare
                                        1554–1616

*Pale death approaches with an equal step, and
knocks indiscriminately at the door of the cottage, and
the portals of the palace.*

Horace
65–8 B.C.

This was a sad way for Mama's life to end. How rapidly
or how slowly would this disease progress?

*Today let me live well; none knows what may be
tomorrow.*

Palladas
400 A.D.

July 1991

Some days were calmer than others, and I would say to
myself, "Oh, this is working out fine. Mama is home. Daddy is
home. Around-the-clock assistance at home is working well.
Daddy and Mama are able to be together in the home they built
together forty-five years ago. Someone is there to cook and
clean for them and to bathe Mama and supervise her in the
bathroom." Other days began with an accident. Mama would
get up and go to the bathroom, and before Daddy or the nursing
assistant could get to her, her bladder or bowels would act.
Diapers didn't always help. Daddy began to call each morning
to report on the situation. The pain of seeing Mama deteriorate
was terrible for Daddy to bear.

Ah, there are moments for us here, when seeing
Life's inequalities, and woe, and care,
The burdens laid upon our mortal being
Seem heavier than the human heart can bear.

Phoebe Cary
1824–1871

How could Mama continue to be cared for at home? Was it time to let the professionals at the nursing home do it? The nursing home became our plan for "taking care of her" in the best way we possibly could. It was becoming apparent that the time was coming closer for Mama to leave the home she had loved and cared for for more than forty-five years. We stopped thinking about what others thought. We didn't emphasize the opinions of others concerning this decision. We did what we felt was right at the time.

Do all the good you can
By all the means you can
In all the ways you can
In all the places you can
At all the times you can
To all the people you can
As long as ever you can.

John Wesley
1703–1791

Since this was not our first exposure to Alzheimer's, we knew what was coming—we just didn't know when. Mama was more like a child than an adult. She was helpless but, unlike a baby, she didn't learn new things or do new things. She continued to lose more and more of herself and her abilities. Her loss was my loss too.

> *No one without experience knows the anguish which*
> *children can cause and yet be loved.*
>> Elisabeth of Braunschweig
>> 1510–1558

Mama was continuing to deteriorate. Some days I adapted. Other days I grieved.

> *Be still sad heart! and cease repining;*
> *Behind the clouds, the sun's still shining;*
> *Thy fate is the common fate of all,*
> *Into each life some rain must fall,*
> *Some days must be dark and dreary.*
>> Henry Wadsworth Longfellow
>> 1807–1882

1992

My mother's youngest sister had been in a nursing home twelve years, and we had watched her deterioration. While in her forties she was diagnosed with brain cancer. Later specialists discovered it was not cancer at all, and in 1992 she died. Her death certificate read: Cause of death, Alzheimer's disease.

As more and more of my family members became lost to Alzheimer's, it didn't take very long for me to figure out that the key to my getting through all of this was going to be the way I dealt with these changes—the way I personally responded. I couldn't change the circumstances, but I could change the way I dealt with them. I vowed to be more hopeful and determined to make a difference. I sought strength beyond myself to deal with this change.

> *But be not thou far from me, O Lord: O my strength,*
> *haste thee to help me.*
>
> Psalms 22:19

We discovered that we were not in control of Mama's behavior. She wasn't either.

> *'Tis hard to smile when one would weep,*
> *To speak when one would silent be;*
> *To wake when one would wish to sleep,*
> *And to wake to agony.*
>
> Anne Hunter
> 1742–1821

A few chuckles along the way helped. There were a few times that Mama was able to chuckle too—but not too often.

One day of smiles happened when we were having a meal together while Mama was still being cared for at home. Mama brought her roll-on deodorant to the table, as she often did. She set it by her plate as if it were a salt or pepper shaker. In the middle of the meal, there was silence around the table and the atmosphere seemed heavy, but my husband broke the silence by asking, "Would someone please pass the deodorant?" Mama kept eating, but the rest of us got a chuckle out of his remark.

> *Some things are of that nature as to make*
> *One's fancy chuckle while his heart doth ache.*
>   Bunyan
>   1628–1688

While Mama was being cared for at home, many longtime friends cooked food and tried to help out. Often they didn't know how to respond to Mama.

> *Forget injuries, never forget kindnesses.*
>   Confucius
>   551–479 B.C.

Alzheimer's disease is a slowly progressing, degenerative brain disease. After diagnosis, victims generally live between two and eight years. Mother was fifty-one years old when we first noticed her early symptoms. She is now seventy-four.

We've watched Alzheimer's impair mother's memory, her judgment, and her ability to function. Who are we to her? We are probably total strangers. Looking into the mirror, Mama would not even be able to recognize her own face. There is still no known cause or cure for this disease.

Learning more about the disease and educating others about it creates within me a sense of usefulness. The latest information that I know of on drugs being designed to treat the four million Americans with Alzheimer's appeared in *U.S.A. Today* in late July, 1998:

> "Drugs designed to treat the four million Americans with Alzheimer's disease fall into three categories," says Steven DeKosky, chairman of the Alzheimer's Association's medical and scientific advisory council and director of the Alzheimer's disease Center at the University of Pittsburgh.
>
> "Some treat symptoms involving memory, attention, concentration, judgment and language, by preserving acetylcholine, a brain chemical that deteriorates in Alzheimer's. Others are aimed at stopping or slowing the progression of disease by various strategies, including reduction of inflammation, thought to be caused by the buildup of amyloid fibrils. Most promising," he says, "are drugs targeted at heading off or reversing that buildup and other processes in the brain that lead to disease."

From the discontent of man,
The world's best progress springs.

Ella Wheeler Wilcox
1855–1919

New treatment methods are continually being tested. Some of the treatments permit the Alzheimer's victim to remain functioning at a higher level for a longer period of time.

Look to this day! For it is life, the very life of life....
For yesterday is already a dream, and tomorrow is only
a vision; but Today, well-lived, makes every yesterday a
dream of happiness, and every tomorrow a vision of
hope.

Sanskrit
1500 B.C.

We knew that eventually Mama would get worse, but we learned to live each day, one day at a time.

...but though our outward man perish, yet the
inward man is renewed day by day.

II Corinthians 4:16

After a few months of this around-the-clock professional care at home for Mama, it was obvious such care was not enough. Daddy's own health was deteriorating, and he was exhausted.

Daddy and I really wanted to keep Mama at home, but the toll on my father was just too much. On one particular day, Daddy and I were home alone because Mama was in the hospital with a kidney infection. So, this very sad morning at breakfast, I said to Daddy, "You know, Daddy, Mama is not herself anymore, but you are still Daddy, and we have to look out for you too. We need to see if one of the rooms we've looked at, at the nursing home, is still available." Both of us, with tears in our eyes, agreed. This decision made at the kitchen table that morning allowed Daddy to live in the home that he and Mother had built together for another couple of years. But it caused us to take the trip we wished we would never have to make.

August 6, 1991

I drove that day. Mother and Daddy were in the back seat of the car and I was the driver. (I'd been a driver before—one day several years ago for Senator Bob Dole—but this was different.) How could it be? Mother and Daddy sat in the back seat holding hands. Words were not exchanged. In fact, Mother never spoke a word the entire trip. Occasionally Daddy or I would ask her if she was all right and she would nod yes. She didn't appear to be annoyed or happy, or show any emotion. She was pensive. We were sad. We knew that this long drive was another path down that road of long goodbyes. I don't know if she understood that this was a watershed in the development of her illness. Several times we told her that we were taking her where people who knew what they were doing could take care of her. As I looked in the rear-view mirror, I could see her just gazing out the window. Most often Daddy's eyes were on her, and it was obvious to me that this was one of the last times he'd be taking a ride in a car holding her hand and enjoying her companionship. When we reached the nursing home, we pulled up to the carriage entrance. Mother and Daddy stayed in the car, and I went inside to announce our arrival. Soon the director of nursing and a nursing assistant from the wing where Mother had been assigned arrived to greet me. They brought a wheelchair with them and we all went to the car to meet Mother and Daddy. Mother greeted them with a pleasant smile, and got out of the car with assistance from the director. She seated herself in the wheelchair as Daddy and I watched. The director suggested that we give them an hour or so to get her settled in and that we return at that time and bring her clothes and other belongings that were in the trunk of the car. Daddy and I went to a local restaurant for lunch. Our hearts were breaking.

We could hardly eat, but with each bite we reassured ourselves that what we had done for Mama was for the best—but it was very hard. I still get teary-eyed thinking about that day. It was one of those threshold moments when you know you've just taken a very big step—a step you wish you hadn't had to take at all.

So, even then, that feeling of guilt over abandonment crept in.... No matter how much I had done, how much courage I had been able to muster, it was not good enough. It didn't come close to my own personal standards for what I wanted to see happen to Mama and Daddy and me. I was devastated, disappointed, and frustrated. Yet, from the depths of my despair, I came back to my senses and thought to myself, "You know, this is the way Mama wanted it. She told me so." I was seven years old and on those trips from Grandma's house every Sunday afternoon, she would turn to me and say, "Now, Linda, if anything like this ever happens to me, don't change your life to take care of me. Put me away." How those words haunted me, and yet reassured me...

I felt perplexity and pity for Mama.

We first endure, then pity, then embrace.
                                              Alexander Pope
                                              1688–1744

My thoughts and feelings moved back and forth like the cascading branches of a lovely willow tree that once stood in our yard at home. I went to see Mama every day, sometimes more than once a day for the first several weeks she was in the nursing home. I wanted to know that she was being cared for properly, but most of all, I wanted to know if what we had done was the right thing. I felt guilty and confused over whether or not I could have done more. Was this really the best for Mama—or was it best for me?

If some great Power would agree to make me always think what is true and do what is right, on condition of being turned into a sort of clock and wound up every morning before I got out of bed, I should instantly close with the offer.

T. H. Huxley
1825–1895

Chapter Four

About the Nursing Home We Chose

~ ~

About the nursing home we chose...how did we decide?

Long before we thought we needed a nursing home, we looked for comfortable institutions—both in the area where Daddy and Mother lived and in an area where we had lived and thought we would eventually live again. Since we were familiar with both places, we thought exploring them would give us a good indication of what was available. I also looked at some nursing homes in the Washington, D.C., location where my husband and I were living at the time, but since we couldn't quite bring ourselves to think of moving Mother and Daddy that far from their own roots, I never thought the nursing homes I found there were serious alternatives. Besides, we had no idea how long either of our positions would keep us in the D.C. area.

We were on a waiting list for our first choice nursing home in North Carolina for over a year and only moved up two slots—a frustrating distance from the top of the list and admission for Mama. So, as the time approached for us to confirm the decision to move Mama into a suitable situation, we had to review our choices. We ended up with our number two choice—but with hindsight it turned out to be the best choice. How did we rate the institutions we investigated? What were some of the things that were important to us?

When we were ready to "give up," both emotionally and physically, and say that we just couldn't care for Mama at home any more—we were not caring for her as well as we should be, and her health and safety were more important than our personal preferences—we came to the irrevocable conclusion that we needed a skilled nursing facility.

We came to this conclusion because Mother...

- required help in feeding, bathing, and dressing.
- had lost control of her bladder and bowels. She needed to be diapered.
- was unstable on her feet, and thus required assistance in walking. It was dangerous for her to walk on her own.
- babbled, so you couldn't understand her words. She could not carry on a conversation, and usually was not even able to give simple yes or no answers.
- did not respond to sounds. We wondered if she could hear, but often she would respond to her own name, so we felt that her hearing was not impaired; she was just

not processing what she heard.
- had not attempted to read anything for several months, but we believed her vision was not impaired. She responded to our smiles and our kindness to her.
- may have understood instructions, but often she did not respond to them, so we believed her mental capacity had diminished to the point where she was incapable of doing so.
- required constant supervision and some form of restraint for her own safety. We certainly didn't want her to fall again and suffer another broken hip.
- needed medications, so she required special nursing care.

Once we looked closely at what Mother actually needed, we were able to begin the process of screening nursing homes. That brought about other considerations for us. The first priority was a facility that was close to the home where Mother and Daddy had lived for over forty-five years. If a suitable home could not be found there, the next choice was a home near me. We asked a lot of friends and acquaintances about what they had heard about nursing homes in the area. Initially, we started with a "word of mouth" list. We only considered facilities that had skilled nursing care, which narrowed the list considerably. We drew up a list of six skilled-nursing homes and decided to visit each one.

At first the task of looking at these nursing homes seemed overwhelming, but prior to and during our visit to the first home,

Daddy and I made up a list of the things that were important for us. We discussed the advantages and disadvantages of segregation of the Alzheimer's patients with the officials at each home we visited. Some facilities had a dedicated floor or wing for the Alzheimer's patients, and others did not. Some homes had waiting lists; others did not. We found it useful to ask about the types of certification and deficiencies found in their last state assessment. We wanted to know about complaints from family members and how they were handled. It is important to know if the home accepts Medicare and Medicaid reimbursement. Even though there may be long term care insurance coverage or private funds at the time of entrance, there may be a time in the future when the resident will run out of funds and would need to use these benefits. Cost was a major consideration, so we asked about the monthly charges and how they were broken down. Were there additional charges for services such as laundry, diapers, medications, and other necessities?

Nothing can tell the story quite like a tour of a nursing home. We felt it important to have an official tour of the facility. I had been with a friend when she was visiting her loved one, so I was already familiar with some of the things we would learn on an official tour. Those visits with my friend gave me a first-hand view of what life was like on a daily basis. The planned official tours were also instructive, but the personal visit gave me an opportunity to talk at length with nursing staff and other residents. Daddy and I weighed heavily our own personal impressions of what we observed. We were looking for quality in many different aspects of the home, but primarily interested in safety, comfort, livability, and personnel.

Here are some things we considered on each tour:

Building and Grounds
- Overall condition—clean and neat?
- Well-maintained buildings?
- Emergency exits well marked?
- Handrails for hallways?
- Wheelchair ramps?
- Surrounding neighborhood safe?
- Area where residents could be outside?
- Nice lobby or visiting area?
- Hallways wide enough for two gurney chairs to pass?
- Unpleasant odors?
- Spacious indoor recreation area?
- Comfortable in terms of temperature control?

Resident Rooms
- Well-lighted, clean, neat, with memorabilia present?
- Closet space for clothing, shoes, and other belongings?
- Furniture in good repair?
- Furniture provided, or resident's personal furniture encouraged?
- Bathrooms attached to each room?
- Private rooms available?

- Choice of roommates for semi-private rooms?
- Privacy maintained in each room?
- Rooms with a window to the outside?

Personnel
- Nursing staff locations and number of nurses?
- Nursing aids or nursing assistants—number and locations?
- Ration of staff members to residents?
- Staff screening prior to employment—drug testing, criminal background checks?
- Contract services used?
- Percentage of turnover rate in nursing personnel?
- General impression of the person giving the tour?
- Residents, visitors, and personnel treated with courtesy and respect?
- Atmosphere of friendliness and professionalism?
- Personnel in the kitchen wearing hair nets and did they have on plastic gloves?

Resident Care
- Provisions for dental care, podiatric services, hearing aids?
- Pharmacist who monitors records on each resident?
- Ambulance service?

- Specific hospital where residents are taken in an emergency?
- Residents' dining room clean and attractive?
- Copy of current menu offered?
- Residents look clean and well cared for—clean shaven, fingernails clean and trimmed?
- Specific religious and recreational activities offered in the health care unit?
- Number of residents each nursing assistant feeds at meal time?
- Food primarily prepared from fresh, frozen, or canned products?
- Special bathing areas equipped with sturdy lifting devices and safety mechanisms?

I asked to see a sample of the documents I would be asked to sign prior to Mother's entrance into the nursing home. These documents were important. They spelled out the responsibilities that I, as holder of power of attorney for my mother, would assume. They also spelled out the responsibilities that the nursing home would assume. I did not want to hurriedly read and sign such documents on what would be a very emotional day, the day Mother would actually enter the nursing home. I felt it best to review them ahead of time, so that if I had questions I could get them answered prior to Mother's admission.

Policies

- Current state license?
- Physician selected by resident or by facility?
- Staff level authorized to call physician?
- Care plan process explained, and family invited to participate?
- Family members welcome anytime?
- Special policies of the home explained?
- Policies related to smoking?
- Residents' rights and responsibilities information explained?
- Nursing home's policy on restraints?

If any of you lack wisdom, let him ask of God, that giveth to all men liberally, and upbraideth not; and it shall be given him.

James 1:5

There are lots of other questions that one could ask when going through the process I have described. However, the questions most important to me were related to safety, comfort, and quality of care. If we had been looking for placement someplace other than in a skilled nursing facility, there would have been many other considerations. But since Mother needed skilled care at the time of her placement, that narrowed our list of what we were looking for in a home. The thought that was foremost in my mind at that time was, "I must see things as they are, not as I would like them to be."

The greatest devotion, greater than learning and praying, consists in accepting the world exactly as it happens to be.

Hasidic saying

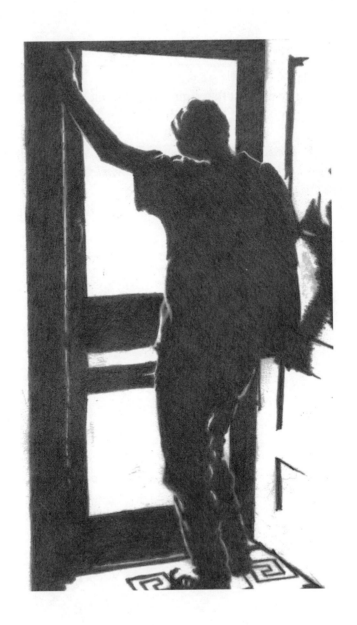

Chapter Five

Now, Dad's a Lonely Heart

~ ~

L ife at home without Mama was lonely and empty for Daddy. He endured that new lifestyle for two years until his health deteriorated, and then he went to live in the same nursing home as Mama.

> *But who can count the beatings of the lonely heart?*
> Susan Edmonstone Ferrier
> 1782–1854

"Home is not home without your mama," Daddy would often say after Mama went to live at the nursing home.

> *'Tis sad to think the days are gone,*
> *When those we love were near;*

I sit upon this mossy stone,
and sigh when none can hear.

Anne Home
1742–1821

Daddy woke to silence, aloneness. He went to bed with silence and coldness. Without Mama, his familiar house was suddenly quite unfamiliar.

Ah, me, what can please or cheer one who has no
hope of happiness in life? Solitude and amusement from
external objects is all I hope for; home is the abyss of
misery!

Elizabeth Holland
1771–1845

One of Daddy's favorite expressions was, "Nothing in life is certain except change." How right he was. Even he didn't anticipate the kinds of changes Mama's illness would actually bring to our family.

There is certain relief in change, even though it be
from bad to worse; as I have found in travelling in a
stagecoach, that it is often a comfort to shift one's
position and be bruised in a new place.

Washington Irving
1783–1859

Going through massive change, meeting challenges and overcoming adversities in my own personal life, caused me to do a great deal of thinking and caused me to go through a great deal of introspection. Expressions like these came to mind almost hourly... Will I survive all this? Can I make it through this?

The Lord is my rock, and my fortress, and my deliverer; my God, my strength, in whom I will trust...
Psalms 18:2

I realized that it was all right to be annoyed or even feel displeasure, but not all right to let those feelings overtake and control me.

Gold is tried by fire, brave men by adversity.
Seneca
6–65 A.D.

Some days I couldn't believe this was actually happening to me and my family. For the first time in my life I felt so isolated, thrust into a totally unknown environment, not knowing were to turn for advice, help, or sympathy. My source of strength became what I could draw from my past, from my roots and upbringing, and what I found daily on my own through my reading, prayer, and study. I relied more and more on this special strength.

The Lord is my strength and my shield; my heart trusted in him and I am helped.

Psalms 28:7

Chapter Six

A House of Dreams

~ ~

Our home was very special. It was Mama and Daddy's lifelong gift to one another. Daddy cut the timber himself, laid the brick foundation, and put up every board. Mama's decorative touches—even her hand-painted trim on the fireplace—elicit special memories. The three of us moved into that home when I was five months old, and I moved out when I got married. That home truly was a house of dreams for our small family.

> *A house of dreams untold,*
> *It looks out over the whispering treetops*
> *And faces the setting sun.*
>
> Edward Macdowell
> 1861–1908

Mama and Daddy loved their life together in the house where they had lived since Thanksgiving Day in 1946.

Those gifts are ever the most acceptable which the giver has made precious.

Ovid
43 B.C.

When I visited Daddy, I too noticed the emptiness in the house without Mama. Signs of her once happy life in their home were everywhere—lovely handmade draperies in the living room and dining room, the handmade quilted coverlets in each bedroom, and her fine china placed perfectly in the china cabinet.

Stop and consider! Life is but a day.

Keats
1795–1821

Outside, Mama's rose bushes bloomed. She could no longer walk by and admire their beauty.

There's not a wind but whispers of thy name;
And not a flow'r that grows beneath the moon,
But in its hues and fragrance tells a tale
Of thee, my love.

Barry Cornwall
1787–1874

The pear and apple trees continued to bear fruit, as did the blackberry bushes and the grapevines. But there wouldn't be any more of Mama's pies or preserves.

> *Now it is gone—our brief hours travel past,*
> *Each with its thought or deed its why or how;*
> *But know each parting hour gives up a ghost*
> *To dwell within thee—an eternal now!*
>
> Coleridge
> 1772–1834

I wanted to walk into the house and see Mama crocheting again, or sitting at her sewing machine, or in the kitchen cooking again.

> *One today is worth two tomorrows.*
>
> Benjamin Franklin
> 1706–1790

I walked over to the vanity table in the bedroom. There was a skein of crochet thread with her crochet hook resting in the thread. I picked it up. It was like picking up a piece of Mama's yesterday. I longed for the times that this thread represented. I longed to be with Mama again.

> *No cord or cable can so forcible draw, or hold so*
> *fast, as love can do with only a twined thread.*
>
> Robert Burton
> 1577–1640

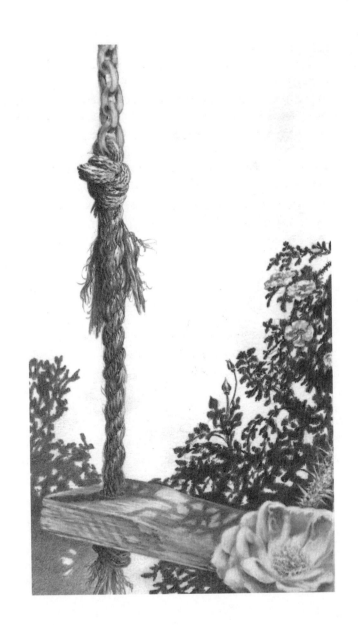

Just outside the kitchen window stand two large oak trees. When I was a girl, these trees were just right for a swing. Daddy made me a sturdy swing with a chain and a handcrafted seat, sanded smooth. Each afternoon when the weather was nice, I would swing high and low. I could see Mama through the kitchen window preparing dinner. I would swing until I was exhausted. I did a lot of thinking in that swing. As I would swing high, my feet would come out over Mama's pink rose bush. Each spring as the roses bloomed, it was beautiful to swing over them and look down on the bees and the blossoms. I went back to that place not long ago. The swing was gone, but I stood and looked over the top of the roses. They looked the same. I smelled the fragrance and it was still fabulously familiar. There was no one at the kitchen window. Mama was gone.

> *When I forget that the stars shine in air,*
> *When I forget that beauty is in stars,*
> *Shall I forget thy beauty.*
>
> James Thomson
> 1700–1748

Mama doesn't stand at the sink in the kitchen and look out the double windows at her beautiful rose bush. She doesn't walk in the garden anymore. Mama doesn't live there any more. Neither do I. Neither does Daddy. We are still saying goodbye.

See the descending sun
Scatt'ring his beams about him as he sinks,
And gilding heaven above...

Gerard Manley Hopkins
1844–1889

Chapter Seven

Ongoing Care

~ ~

I feel it's important to continually assess quality, comfort, and safety issues. Mama needs me now to be her voice, her advocate. If I find things I don't like at the nursing home, I ask the head nurse about them. Problems have almost always been resolved immediately. If they are not, then I proceed up the ladder in the chain of command. I believe I am fair about my own expectations. I do what I am capable of doing for Mama.

No one is useless in this world who lightens the burden of it for anyone else.

Charles Dickens
1812–1870

I frequently expect too much of myself.

*It is a folly to expect men to do all that they may
reasonably be expected to do.*

> Richard Whately
> 1787–1863

What are fair expectations? If there is an issue relating to
Mother's comfort, safety, health, or the quality of her care, I
will definitely speak up. But if I see another resident occasionally wearing a pair of Mother's socks, or one of her blouses
that's gotten mixed up, for example, will I make an issue of it?
No. That alone does not matter that much. It does not affect
Mother's comfort, health, or safety unless the other resident is
wearing socks and Mother is not wearing any at all—or ones
that do not fit, for example. If this mix-up happened more than
once in a while I would think that it could reflect a quality-of-
care issue.

I am sometimes tired and overwhelmed. I often feel a
desire to be set free of this situation.

*A merry heart goes all the day,
A sad tires in a mile.*

> Shakespeare
> 1564–1616

Visiting during different times of the day and visiting
frequently can help me to make these continuing assessments

and judgments about quality of care. Active participation on my part at the home helps me to assure that we are getting and giving the best care possible for Mother.

It's difficult to manage this situation all the time.

Let every dawn of the morning be to you as the beginning of life.
And let every setting of the sun be to you as its close.
Then let every one of these short lives leave its sure record of some kindly thing done for others, some good strength or knowledge gained for yourself.

John Ruskin
1819–1900

During the first couple of years Mother was in the nursing home, she was quite frenetic and agitated. She was totally inattentive, did not respond to hugs and kisses, engaged in loud yelling almost constantly, and did not utter an understandable word. Her conversation consisted only of nonsense words and babbling. This was a very difficult period of time for her, but it was also a difficult time for me. This was not the situation I had hoped for at this time in my life. I was disappointed. We were so united as a family. Now we were all separated.

When lilacs last in the dooryard bloom'd
And the great star early droops in the western sky in
the night,
I mourn'd and yet shall mourn with ever-returning
spring.

Walt Whitman
1819–1892

Every visit with Mama brought me face to face with reality. I looked at her and saw a look of frustration, anxiety, and suffering. I looked into Mama's face and usually saw a tormented expression. This tormented look took its toll on her beautiful skin and marked her smooth, youthful face with lines and wrinkles. Other times I examined her face and saw a subtle smile. During all of these times I wondered what she was thinking—or if she could still think. I saw those same beautiful blue eyes that used to look at me with such love and joy. I wondered what her eyes were seeing when they looked at me now.

It is better to have loved and lost
Than never to have loved at all.

Tennyson
1809–1892

Even today, with Mother being in the nursing home for over seven years, my heart often hopes that Mama doesn't realize what is happening to her, but my mind accepts the fact that she may.

Hope, like the gleaming taper's light
Adorns and cheers our way
And still as darker grows the night
Emits a brighter ray.

Oliver Goldsmith
1730–1774

When I look at Mama, I question what kind of pain she is in—or whether or not she is in any pain at all. I hope not. Part of me realizes that Mama has to endure this pain and suffering on her own. Oh, how I wish I could help.

The thought,
The deadly thought of solitude.

Keats
1795–1821

Here I am face to face with reality again—with each and every visit, each and every moment. Each time I look at Mama I see only a part of the person she once was. This forces me to say goodbye again and again and again....

These, then are my last words to you: Be not afraid
of life. Believe that life is worth living and your belief
will help create the fact.

William James
1842–1910

During those early nursing home years, it was hard to find the good in all of this. It was hard to find the good and the wonderfulness in what remained of Mama. There was so much that was lost, and her yelling and loud demeanor made what I saw of her appear to be so unlovely. So, I just looked at her and wondered, "Mama, where are you?" Mama was gone. I tried not to focus on what was lost, but instead sought out and cherished what remained.

There are some men and women in whose company we are always at our best. All the best stops in our nature are drawn out, and we find music in our souls never felt before.

William Henry Drummond
1854–1907

During Mother's first couple of years in the nursing home, I took the opportunity to do a lot of reading, writing, and talking to others about the hope of new treatments for this terrible disease. I truly needed hope. I kept notes about my thoughts on dealing with this situation, and eventually wrote the first edition of this book, released in 1994, entitled *A Long Goodbye, Reflections on Dealing with Alzheimer's*. This process of reflection and study gave me the information, comfort, and support I needed. It helped me to realize that the progression of Mama's illness is only partially predictable. I must take life one day at a time and be prepared for what happens next.

We must be satisfied to advance in life as we walk—
step by step.

Samuel Smiles
1812–1904

During this time of extensive research and study, I had read about one new drug therapy treatment, tacrine. On Thanksgiving Day, 1993, Mama's physician (who was also at the nursing home on that day) and I discussed administering the drug tacrine. It had only been on the market a couple of months, and while Mama's physician was not overly optimistic because she was not an apparent candidate for the drug, he was willing to try it. So, Mama's treatment began the next week. Her positive response to tacrine gave us some wonderful times together that I do not believe we would otherwise have had. I savored small, infrequent, joyous moments with Mama. These moments joined my fond memories with true reality.

Dost thou love life?
Then do not squander time, for that is the stuff life is
made of.

Benjamin Franklin
1706–1790

I reminded myself that my life was not constantly filled with good things; neither was it filled with all bad.

There is not a heart but has its moments of longing,
yearning for something better, nobler, holier than it
knows now.

Henry Ward Beecher
1813–1887

Initially, Mother's results with tacrine were so dramatic that my husband began taking video clips of our normal visits. He started taking these video clips about two weeks after the drug therapy first began. He ended up with more than fourteen hours of video, and it was so wonderful to see on video, as well as in person, some of the things Mama recaptured. Never did we anticipate that these videos—or clips of them—would be shared outside our family, but I have shared them with professionals who are trying to help families like ours and patients like Mother deal with the disease. Even today, when physicians see these video clips, many of them tell me that they are reminded in a vivid way that their work each and every day does translate into specific help for others. I have learned how important it is to solicit advice and guidance from others when necessary. I've also learned how important it is to be able to give advice to others.

Help thy brother's boat across the river and, lo!
Thine own has reached the shore.

Hindu proverb

One day as I was leaving from my visit with Mama, she waved goodbye. This was the first time she had responded in this way in over two years.

> *No man or woman of the humblest sort can really be*
> *strong, gentle, pure and good without somebody being*
> *helped and comforted by the very existence of goodness.*
>   Phillips Brooks
>   1835–1892

When other family members viewed the video clips we made of our visits with Mother, they told me that they were reminded of hope. The hope represented in the photos we took was the hope that there would someday be a treatment, and even a cure for this disease. This hope helped to eliminate some of the fear. But even today, I fear for myself and my husband that I'm next in line to get the sickness. First Grandma, then Mama—am I next?

> *He has not learned the lesson of life who does not*
> *each day surmount a fear.*
>   Ralph Waldo Emerson
>   1803–1882

I will find additional hopes and dreams because of this illness.

Little minds are tamed and subdued by misfortune,
but great minds rise above it.

Washington Irving
1783–1859

The following are some of the things that were important to us that Mother recaptured as a result of the drug:

- She could once again recognize her own name.
- She could answer questions appropriately with a yes or no answer.
- She could give us hugs and kisses.
- She caught a balloon on her seventieth birthday.
- She said my name once more.
- She asked me some questions.
- She smiled.
- She once again showed her personality by making an emphatic and amusing response from time to time.

So, why were these events important? Before she went on tacrine, she had not smiled, hugged us, or given us a kiss in more than two years. By recapturing those things, we regained a bit of Mother—even if for only a brief moment at a time. Being able to communicate again in only these simple ways had such a positive effect on her and on us.

One of these times of simple pleasure that was captured on video was a day when my husband and I were visiting and she looked up at me and said, "Was your hair brown?" You should have heard me (now a blonde from a bottle) trying to answer that. "Yes, it was brown, but it's blonde now isn't it?" From that I concluded that you can't get away with anything with your mother—not even coloring your hair! Her question was totally initiated by her, and it was shocking and remarkable to me that this woman, who had not started any conversation in two years, would break the silence with such a thoughtful question.

Now to the casual observer, our delight in these simple pleasures may seem truly overstated. However, they were quite significant to Mother, to me, to my dad, and to other family members.

One of the other significant things the drug therapy brought back was a pleasant part of Mother that we had not seen in two years. She went from being combative and loud to sweet and loving again.

This was also significant to Mother's "hands-on care-givers"—those health care workers in the nursing home who cared for Mother day in and day out. They told me how much it meant to them to be greeted by a hug, a kiss, and a smile in the morning instead of a combative, insulting woman.

We enjoyed Mother's partial renewal for about a year. Then Alzheimer's, as it marched along, began to move at an even faster pace. The disease overshadowed the positive effects that the tacrine treatment could offer. Sadly, after about twenty-four months of medication, we discontinued it. At this time Alzheimer's continues winning the race with Mother.

What are the treatments?

The treatments that have been approved by the Food and Drug Administration for treatment of Alzheimer's disease at this time are the following:

- tacrine hydrochloride (a.k.a Cognex® released in 1993)
- donepezil hydrochloride (a.k.a. Aricept® released in 1996)

Both of these medications must be prescribed by a physician and are specifically designed to treat symptoms commonly associated with mild to moderate Alzheimer's disease. These two treatments represent hope. For some people they represent some additional control. Just as the disease affects people in different ways, the treatments may also have different effects and results. Some patients may show no change or improvement in their symptoms. Others may benefit and be able to perform some of the tasks that they have not been able to do for quite some time. These decisions about what is needed, results of treatments, and expectations, vary with each individual and are very personal. Decisions about medications are best left to patient, caregiver, and physician. We were blessed through our experience because it represented a glimmer of hope.

The flowers of all the tomorrows are in the seeds of today.

Chinese proverb

I continue to meet new friends. Many of these friends' interests center around a mutual concern—Alzheimer's.

A friend loveth at all times…
                                        Proverbs 17:17

The good times my family and I experienced with Mother represent hope—they represent the hope of knowing that there are people who care enough to find and release treatments that do offer help and hope, and someday, maybe, there will even be a cure. This treatment and others like it which are either on the market now, or soon will be, are only a start. But it is a start, and I'm thankful that it is being built upon.

There will be times in the next several years that my own dream and vision of a treatment and cure for Alzheimer's will be tested. But, I am thankful that my family had such a positive experience with one therapy and I am eager to move on and build upon that positive experience. I know that my family's story can be a catalyst of inspiration to help others. We are all just beginning to find ways to help one another. So, there truly is help and there is hope.

Our long goodbye continues—and you may have your own long goodbye right now, but you have the power in your hands to offer some comfort, help, and hope. You can use your power to punctuate that long goodbye with an improved quality of life that would not be possible without the care, dedication, and hope you can give.

My family's story is like many stories that could be told by those who read this book. You see your own loved one—you see yourself—coping with this long goodbye. So, we share a common experience. All of these years—in fact, all of my entire life—the disease has tried to destroy my trust and hope in the future. But it can't do it, because of the many others who share my hope and continue to give all the help, love, and warmth that can be given.

Therefore my heart is glad, and my glory rejoiceth:
my flesh also shall rest in hope.

Psalms 16:8

1993

As I said earlier, because of declining health, Daddy went to live in the nursing home where Mother is living. It was hard for him to leave the home he and Mother had built, and where they had lived for over forty-five years, but it was not the same home without Mama.

Daddy had been through World War II, and he was a survivor. Now he was going through another war—a war within himself—and with a disease we know as Alzheimer's. For the rest of his life he will recall some of the sights, sounds, images, and stresses he experienced while dealing with Mother. Sometimes it doesn't take much to bring back all the memories he would just as soon forget, just like with World War II. But with time, the intensity of the memories moderates. Leaving the house where those memories were generated would not remove them, but it was certain to place them at a distance.

We simply closed the house, left the sugar bowl on the table, left everything in place and made it clear to Daddy that if he didn't like his "second home," he could come back to his "first one." We talked a lot about the decision before we made it, and about others he knew who had second homes—at the coast or in the mountains. Seen in that light, the nursing home, with Mama close, could be his second home. He could go and visit Mama anytime he wanted to, and he wouldn't be giving up anything. This solution gave Daddy a strong feeling of personal security and helped to bolster his attitude and defenses about giving up so much at one time. His new home would permit him to engage in different activities with different people like him, who were looking for other connections. Also, his new home would give Daddy an opportunity to reflect, if he chose to do so, on the life he and Mother had together, what his life had meant to the community where he lived, on the church where he was so active, and on the beliefs and commitments that he held so dear.

Friends and family came frequently to visit with Daddy and Mama. Making the one-hundred-mile trip took a great deal of commitment on their part, and their visits were always appreciated. Fellow deacons from the church where Daddy had been so active were free and open with comments about how much Daddy and Mother had meant to the church family. Being able

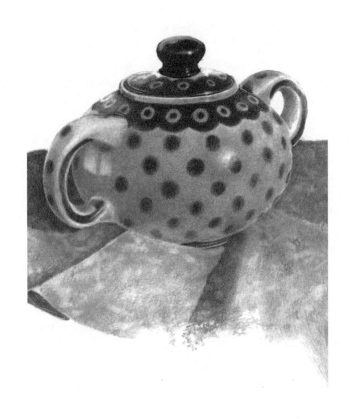

to look back on these good parts of his past life was a positive experience for Daddy, and the visits were truly cherished.

Daddy adjusted, but he sometimes grieved about his own deteriorating condition. He still has difficulty accepting his "new self." He still grieves about Mother and her condition. Despite the idea of a new era for him, it's hard for him to accept his "new self" and his new surroundings. It's hard for him to find ways to be "valued" as he once was or to recognize how much quality of life he still maintains.

I continue to see Daddy diminish in physical, psychological, and emotional ways, and it's difficult for him to express his thoughts, feelings, and emotions. But I trust that he still experiences the gift of life—the gift of the promise of life beyond us...the spiritual connectedness each of us, alone, can sense, feel, and live.

One thing I have experienced in "getting beyond" Mother's illness is the gift of connectedness—going beyond ourselves, reaching out to others, and through my own spirituality, reaching out to the Lord. I am now better able to accept the limitations of my own physical self and concentrate more on my spiritual bonding with God. Maintaining a balance between my own spiritual and physical self is a conscious and continuous effort. But as I achieve more and more of this balance, fear and anxiety seem to disappear, and I am able to make the most of each day and of each moment of each day.

Connectedness makes me feel more in control. I can control the way I feel about Mama's sickness and the way I choose to respond to my own thoughts, feelings, and emotions about it. I am not a victim. In fact, I am blessed with the strength and courage to get beyond this disease and beyond myself.

The Lord will give strength...

Psalms 29:11

Another aspect of the connectedness I experience is a more intense appreciation for the beautiful things around me. A walk in the woods, in the garden, or on the beach is such a special event. I am better able to sense beauty in sights, smells, and sounds at such marvelous places. I appreciate things more because I see how rapidly they can be taken away.

...the earth is full of the goodness of the Lord.

Psalms 33:5

Chapter Eight

The Final Goodbye

~ ~

Dying is one thing—death is yet another. Alzheimer's has helped me to come to grips, although in my case quite slowly, with both of these issues. I refer to both a long goodbye and a final goodbye. Most of this book has dealt with the long goodbye, but all of us who deal with the long goodbye must also eventually deal with the final goodbye. Alzheimer's disease is a terminal illness. Various systems and organs in the body are failing—it leads to a state of dying and no treatments have yet proven to be effective against it. Death of the body is usually attributed to complications relating to Alzheimer's. But, in the final analysis, death is brought about by the Alzheimer's disease itself.

I am sad that Mama is unable to lead a complete, full, and satisfying life.

A feeling of sadness and longing,
That is not akin to pain,
And resembles sorrow only
as the mist resembles the rain.

Henry Wadsworth Longfellow
1807–1882

    Mother, as an Alzheimer's patient, does not have the opportunity to say farewell through either her words or her actions. Unlike some other illnesses where there is a period of time when the body may be failing but the mental capacities are still functioning, this is not the case with an Alzheimer's patient. Therefore, Mother and her family and friends are not given an opportunity to work through grief together preceding the final goodbye. The special connectedness through communication is missing. A great separation exists even before death. I choose to see this living separation as a preparation for the ultimate total separation from Mama. I accept these changes taking place in my life and hers, and I anticipate that there will be even more change.

No longer forward nor behind
I look in hope or fear
But grateful, take the good I find
The best of now and here.

John Greenleaf Whittier
1807–1892

Because of my faith, however, I do not feel that this separation will be final. Our bodies will separate, but I believe that our spiritual connectedness will continue through memories, teachings, and values we have shared. The spiritual connection will last, not just through my lifetime, but for eternity.

I often wish that Alzheimer's disease victims had a special hospice available just for this illness. The support system offered by Hospice is so strong, and the services offered are so supportive to the family as well as to the loved one. The dignity and respect for human life is so evident in the work they do. They provide emotional, religious, and spiritual support at a time when this is much needed. In the case of Alzheimer's disease or other dementia-related illnesses, the timespan during which these services are needed is often much longer than what the support system is designed to offer. Therefore, many families who are in need of consolation and support do not ever get them.

In God is my salvation and my glory: the rock of my strength, and my refuge, is in God.
                                                    Psalms 62:7

Chapter Nine

Me Dealing with Me

~ ~

S ometimes "me dealing with me" was as difficult as me dealing with Mama and her disease. My thoughts fluctuated from believing I was dealing with the situation in a very intelligent, capable, and mature way and realizing that I was grieving from the reality of the situation. I learned that I did have choices. I could choose to cope, or I could choose to change. I chose to take control of my life and make some changes.

We are what we repeatedly do.

Aristotle
384–322 B.C.

At times I felt depression, anger, guilt, shame, loneliness, helplessness, and denial, but I didn't let my thoughts dwell on those feelings. I replaced those feelings by thinking more comforting thoughts.

Dream manfully and nobly and thy dreams shall be prophets.
Edward George Bulwer-Lytton
1803–1873

At times I also felt pain, sorrow, fear, anxiety, frustration, self-pity, annoyance, displeasure, irritation, and rage. I quickly substituted thoughts that were more uplifting, and those thoughts changed my feelings.

Thoughts are but dreams until their effects be tried.
Shakespeare
1564–1616

I endured all of this change.

I'll not willingly offend, nor be easily offended:
What's amiss I'll strive to mend, And endure what can't be mended.
Isaac Watts
1674–1748

Often others asked me to describe the hardest aspects of dealing with Alzheimer's disease. I usually described the following things:

Mama losing control of her bladder, and thus her deportment as a cultured woman; dealing with the loss of her beautiful personality; aching for the lost communication with her. These were and still are the most difficult aspects of the sickness for me.

True courage consists not in flying from the storms of life, but in braving and steering through them with prudence.
Hannah Webster Foster
1758–1840

As each of Mama's physical and mental characteristics drifted away, I grieved for each one because that part of her was gone forever.

The man who removes a mountain begins by carrying away small stones.
Chinese proverb

Birthdays were always very special at our house. In my earliest remembrances, Mama always baked a cake for my birthday and for Daddy's. Certain birthdays were celebrated with just the three of us—but others included extended family or friends. I recall my sixth birthday as a surprise party with many of my friends. But one of the most special parts of every birthday were the conversations. This was a time Mama used to

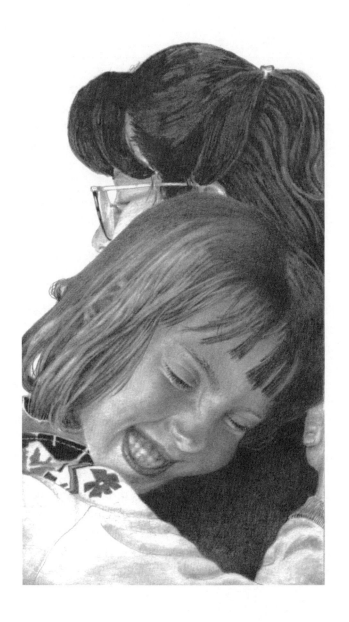

tell me how very remarkable it was for her to have me as a daughter. She would tell me how she looked upon me as a "special gift." She never characterized my specialness in a way that made me feel superior—just super! In fact, she would always conclude with something such as, "You are no better than anyone else, but you are just as good."

She was so honored to be a parent and took that role very seriously. She would tell me that she felt that this "gift" that she had been given was really a loan, and that she had only a limited time with me—and she treasured each moment. On my birthday in 1993, almost two years after Mother had gone to the nursing home, I realized how much I missed our birthday conversations.

Mama was not Mama anymore. I realized that my most vocal booster, supporter, and cheerleader was gone. She was no longer able to tell me how precious I was to her, how much she loved me, how much confidence she had in me, how I could do anything I wanted to do if I worked hard enough and wanted it badly enough...

All that I am or hope to be, I owe to my angel mother.

Abraham Lincoln
1809–1865

She was not the mother I once knew. As she changed, I changed too.

Grief knits two hearts in closer bonds than happiness ever can; and common sufferings are far stronger links than common joys.

Lamartine
1790–1869

Visits in the nursing home can be very special. Below are some of the things I have learned that make visits even more special:

- taking a treat that we can eat together—such as soft ice cream.
- taking a tape recorder and playing some very soft, soothing music.
- taking a stroll together, with Mama in the wheelchair.
- taking the staff something—a plate of cookies or fruit.
- just being together...holding hands...not feeling I have to entertain her.

Often I say to Mama: "I'm Linda. I'm your daughter. I'm here with you. I love you. Everything is all right."

Life is made up, not of great sacrifices or duties, but of little things, in which smiles and kindness and small obligations, given habitually are what win and preserve the heart and secure comfort.

Sir Humphry Davy
1778–1829

Sometimes her beautiful blue eyes look into my eyes and say, "I understand." Sometimes they don't.

Not much talk, a great sweet silence.
                                        Henry James
                                        1811–1882

It is within my power to guide my thoughts and my activities.

It has been my observation that people are just about as happy as they make up their minds to be.
                                        Abraham Lincoln
                                        1809–1865

There are always adjustments that we must make when adversity strikes. There are adjustments we must make when positive things happen to us as well. So, I can't let this situation control my entire life. I have to remind myself that I have my own identity and persona, and that my identity and position in life are not totally derived from Mama and Daddy.

Think from whence thou camest, and blush;
Where thou art, and sigh;
and tremble to remember whither thou shalt go.
                                        Elizabeth Grymeston
                                        1563–1603

When bad things happen to us, we often pause and say something like, "Why me? Why is this happening to me?" Do we ask this when good things happen to us as well? Who knows why this disease happened to Mama. It just did. It is possible to learn from this situation.

Impossible is a word only to be found in the dictionary of fools.

Napoleon
1769–1821

Getting beyond all the pain and grief of dealing with the disease is very important to me. However, there are still times when something triggers a past memory or event. Small distinctive impressions transport me back to a past that I still long for. I recently heard someone beside me in a dress shop remark about the fabric and workmanship of a garment. I thought for a brief moment that it was Mama, only to look over and see that it wasn't.

No man is free who is not a master of himself.

Epictetus
60–120 A.D.

As we were singing a familiar hymn one Sunday in church, I noticed that the lady standing beside me was singing alto. Those familiar words and notes were the very same ones Mama used to sing when she stood beside me in church.

Joy descends gently upon us like the evening dew,
and does not patter down like a hail storm.

Johann Richter
1763–1825

I'm a separate person from my Mama. I'm independent, and I'm not responsible for Mama's behavior.

Make the best use of what is in your power, and take
the rest as it happens.

Epictetus
60–120 A.D.

I tolerate my own sadness over this situation.

They can conquer who believe they can.

John Dryden
1631–1700

I do not totally relinquish my own ambitions in order to give exclusive attention to Mama.

Make the most of yourself, for this is all there is of
you.

Ralph Waldo Emerson
1803–1882

Just when I think that I've gotten accustomed to Mama's illness, some new change occurs in her, and I grieve all over again.

The longer we dwell on our misfortunes the greater is their power to harm us.

Voltaire
1694–1778

I won't let this disease prevent me from realizing my own hopes and dreams.

The winds and waves are always on the side of the ablest navigators.

Edward Gibbon
1737–1794

I am thankful for each new day, and I work daily to enrich my own future.

The wise man will make more opportunities than he finds.

Francis Bacon
1561–1626

I am grateful that I have the opportunity to develop new interests for myself.

Happiness depends upon ourselves.

Aristotle
4th Century B.C.

I have control of my own life, and I can change it through my thoughts and actions.

Victory belongs to the most persevering.

Napoleon
1769–1821

The future most likely holds some very painful, emotional times, but I will handle those times when they come—not today.

Man, like the bridge, was designed to carry the load of the moment, not the combined weight of a year at once.

William A. Ward
1812–1882

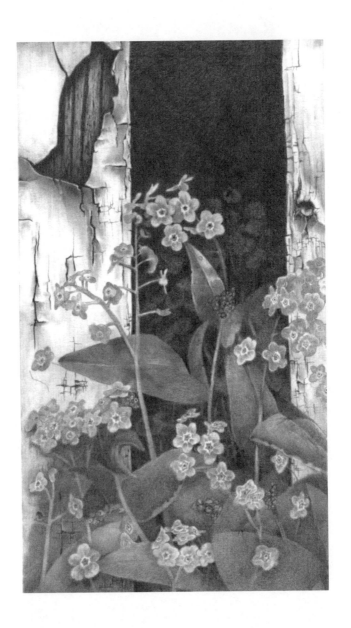

Chapter Ten

Helping Myself by Helping Others

~ ~

During the past several years when I have been called upon to talk with other caregivers, the following dilemmas have seemed to come up most frequently. I encourage caregivers, family members, and friends to keep notes on creative approaches that work for them in handling various situations. I encourage you to do the same and share your ideas and creative solutions with others who are going through their own long goodbyes. This section is provided as a model for your own record of those ideas. If something helped you or your loved one, it will most likely help others also. So, use this section to write down those ideas. Share your strength by giving it away. Help yourself by helping others.

- What I have found to be effective in handling mood changes in my loved one.

- What I have done when my loved one appears to be living in the past.

- How I have dealt with my Alzheimer's patient's feeding at mealtime.

- What methods I have found to help the main caregiver take a break from looking after the patient.

- What caused me to know that it was no longer safe for the Alzheimer's patient to live at home.

- What I have done in my community to encourage increased availability of assistance for caregivers who have Alzheimer's patients at home.

- What I have learned about giving medications or not giving medications to control the Alzheimer's patient's behavior.

- What I have learned that is the most significant thing I can do to help my Alzheimer's patient.

- What I believe is the most clear-cut evidence that the memory loss being experienced by my loved one is truly Alzheimer's disease.

- What I have learned about a possible cure for this disease.

- What I have learned about when the actual onset of this disease took place in my loved one.

- What I have learned about life expectancy following diagnosis of this disease.

- What I have learned about dealing with an Alzheimer's patient from a caregiver perspective.

- What I have learned about the appropriate time to move an Alzheimer's patient to a nursing home.

- What important guidelines I have learned relative to safety and happiness when dealing with an Alzheimer's patient.

- What I have learned that can help family and friends accept and pull together in working with the Alzheimer's patient.

- What I have learned about the medications that are currently on the market for Alzheimer's disease.

- What I have learned about the early signs of Alzheimer's.

- What I have learned about the role genetics plays in Alzheimer's.

- What I have learned about any measures to take to prevent Alzheimer's.

- What I have learned that is the most helpful in making nursing home visits more enriching experiences for myself and for my Alzheimer's loved one.

- What I can do for my own physical well-being.

- What I can do for my own emotional well-being.

- What I can do for my own spiritual well-being.

- What I have done to get through and go beyond a long goodbye.

I will go in the strength of the Lord God…
                                        Psalms 71:16

Author's Note

When my friend Jeanette suggested that I put on paper some of my thoughts that I had found useful, she had no idea how this suggestion would grow and be used by others. After reformatting several pages of handwritten notes I had kept over the years, which reflected discussions I had on Alzheimer's with friends, physicians, and relatives, I added some classical quotations that I found instructive, humorous, or consoling. For this edition, I continued by adding biographical information and some more detailed information that I felt captured watershed moments during this journey of our long goodbye.

One of the struggles I dealt with when I first realized that I needed information about Alzheimer's, since my mother was affected by the disease, was that I was too much involved in dealing with my own day-to-day emotions to find time to read the many wonderful, full-length books available on the subject of Alzheimer's. How does one just stop and say, "Hold it! I need more information. I'll continue dealing with Mama later after I've gotten more information."

Obviously that's impossible. Therefore, the format I selected for presentation is designed as brief thoughts, some of which can be read in one sitting, or that can be read as a thought or two each day. There are hundreds of other comments and quotations that could be added by those who have also dealt with this disease. The ones included here are those that have personally helped me the most. My hope and prayer is that they will help you too, as you and your loved ones go through and beyond your own long goodbye.

For additional information on Alzheimer's disease and caregiving, or to find out about a local Alzheimer's support group, contact:

Alzheimer's Association
Suite 1000
919 North Michigan Avenue
Chicago, IL 60611

800-272-3900

How to Contact the Author

Dr. Linda Morrison Combs is a former Assistant Secretary for Management at the U. S. Department of Treasury. She resigned that position to become a caregiver. She is currently a caregiver, speaker, consultant, and author.

To bring her into your company or organization, contact Linda at her office.

Linda's Office
Phone: 336-760-3905 • Fax: 336-760-3855
E-mail: linda@combsmusic.com
Web site: www.combsmusic.com/ALG.html

About the Author

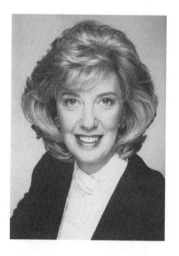

Dr. Linda Combs began her career as a teacher and educator, which led to administrative positions in the Winston-Salem school system and subsequently to management positions, in a bank and in state and federal government. When her reputation as an educator, business manager and public servant came to the attention of the White House, she was appointed by President Reagan to serve as Deputy Undersecretary for Management at the Department of Education and later served as an executive in the Department of Veterans Affairs.

President Bush selected Linda Combs to be Assistant Secretary for Management at the U. S. Department of Treasury; and she was Vice Chair of the President's Council for Management Improvement (PCMI).

Dr. Combs left her government positions to return to North Carolina, where she became the primary caregiver for both her parents, who now require nursing home care. The author lives in Winston-Salem, with her husband, Dave Combs, a composer, inventor, and photographer.